ANESTHESIA, THE HEART AND THE VASCULAR SYSTEM

DEVELOPMENTS IN CRITICAL CARE MEDICINE AND ANESTHESIOLOGY

Prakash, O. (ed.): Applied Physiology in Clinical Respiratory Care. 1982. ISBN 90-247-2662-X.

McGeown, Mary G.: Clinical Management of Electrolyte Disorders. 1983. ISBN 0-89838-559-8.

Scheck, P.A., Sjöstrand, U.H., and Smith, R.B. (eds.): Perspectives in High Frequency Ventilation. 1983. ISBN 0-89838-571-7.

Stanley, T.H., and Petty, W.C. (eds.): New Anesthetic Agents, Devices and Monitoring Techniques. 1983. ISBN 0-89838-566-0.

Prakash, O. (ed.): Computing in Anesthesia and Intensive Care. 1983. ISBN 0-89838-602-0.

Stanley, T.H., and Petty, W.C. (eds.): Anesthesia and the Cardiovascular System. 1984. ISBN 0-89838-626-8.

Van Kleef, J.W., Burm, A.G.L., and Spierdijk, J. (eds.): Current Concepts in Regional Anaesthesia. 1984. ISBN 0-89838-644-6.

Prakash, O. (ed.): Critical Care of the Child. 1984. ISBN 0-89838-661-6.

Stanley, T.H., and Petty, W.C. (eds.): Anesthesiology: Today and Tomorrow. 1985. ISBN 0-89838-705-1.

Rahn, H., and Prakash, O. (eds.): Acid-base Regulation and Body Temperature. 1985. ISBN 0-89838-708-6.

Stanley, T.H., and Petty, W.C. (eds.): Anesthesiology 1986. 1986. ISBN 0-89838-779-5.

de Lange, S., Hennis, P.J., and Kettler, D. (eds.): Cardiac Anaesthesia: Problems and Innovations. 1986. ISBN 0-89838-794-9.

Stanley, T.H., and Petty, W.C. (eds.): Anesthesia, the Heart and the Vascular System. 1987. ISBN 0-89838-851-1.

ANESTHESIA, THE HEART AND THE VASCULAR SYSTEM
Annual Utah Postgraduate Course in Anesthesiology 1987

edited by

THEODORE H. STANLEY, MD
W. CLAYTON PETTY MD

Department of Anesthesiology
The University of Utah Medical School
Salt Lake City
U.S.A.

1987 **MARTINUS NIJHOFF PUBLISHERS**
a member of the KLUWER ACADEMIC PUBLISHERS GROUP
DORDRECHT / BOSTON / LANCASTER

Distributors

for the United States and Canada: Kluwer Academic Publishers, P.O. Box 358, Accord Station, Hingham, MA 02018-0358, USA
for the UK and Ireland: Kluwer Academic Publishers, MTP Press Limited, Falcon House, Queen Square, Lancaster LA1 1RN, UK
for all other countries: Kluwer Academic Publishers Group, Distribution Center, P.O. Box 322, 3300 AH Dordrecht, The Netherlands

Library of Congress Cataloging in Publication Data

ISBN-13: 978-94-010-7979-2   e-ISBN-13: 978-94-009-3295-1
DOI: 10/1007/978-94-009-3295-1

PREFACE

Theodore H. Stanley, M.D.
W. Clayton Petty, M.D.

Anesthesia, the Heart and the Vascular System contains the Refresher
Course manuscripts of the presentations of the 32nd Annual Postgraduate
Course in Anesthesiology which took place at the Westin Hotel Utah
Convention Center in Salt Lake City, Utah, February 20-24, 1987. The
chapters reflect new data and concepts within the general framework of
"risk, preoperative evaluation and monitoring," "cerebral, pulmonary and
peripheral vascular disease," "new agents, their advantages and their
problems" and "pediatric, cardiac and non-cardiac surgery." The purposes
of the textbook are to 1) act as a reference for the anesthesiologists
attending the meeting, and 2) serve as a vehicle to bring many of the
latest concepts in anesthesiology to others within a short time of the
formal presentation. Each chapter is a brief but sharply focused glimpse
of the interests in anesthesia expressed at the conference. This book
and its chapters should not be considered complete treatises on the subjects addressed but rather attempts to summarize the most salient points.
This textbook is the fifth in a continuing series documenting the proceedings of the Postgraduate Course in Salt Lake City. We hope that this
and the past and future volumes reflect the rapid and continuing evolution
of anesthesiology in the late twentieth century.

TABLE OF CONTENTS

Contributing Authors

Arnes, J.F., MD, Department of Anesthesiology, University of Texas Medical
    Branch, Galveston, Texas, USA

Berry, F.A., MD, Department of Anesthesiology, University of Virginia
    Medical Center, Charlottesville, Virginia, USA

Greenley, W.J., MD, Department of Anesthesiology, Duke University Medical
    Center, Durham, North Carolina, USA

Gregory, G.A., MD, Department of Anesthesia, University of California, San
    Francisco, San Francisco, California

Haigs, J.C., BVMS, MSc, Western College of Veterinary Medicine, Department
    Herd Medicine & Theriogenology, University of Saskatchewan, Saskatoon,
    Canada

Katz, R.L., MD, Department of Anesthesiology, UCLA School of Medicine, Los
    Angeles, California, USA

Lange, de, S., MD, Ph D, Department of Anesthesiology, Academisch
    Ziekenhuis, Leiden, The Netherlands

Michenfelder, J.D., MD, Department of Anesthesiology, Mayo Clinic,
    Rochester, Minnesota, USA

Miller, Jr., E.D., MD, Department of Anesthesiology, University of Virginia
    Medical Center, Charlottesville, Virginia, USA

Reiz, S., Ph D, MD, Department of Anesthesiology, Umeå University, Umeå,
    Sweden

Roizen, M.F., MD, Department of Anesthesia & Critical Care, University of
    Chicago Medical Center, Chicago, Illinois, USA

Wong, K.C., MD, Ph D, Department of Anesthesiology, University of Utah
    School of Medicine, Salt Lake City, Utah, USA

Zaiden, J.R., MD, Department of Anesthesiology, Emory University School of
    Medicine, Atlanta, Georgia, USA

DIABETES: PREOPERATIVE EVALUATION AND INTRAOPERATIVE MANAGEMENT

Simon de Lange, M.D.

Diabetes is the commonest endocrine disorder occurring in about 2-3% of the Western population. It has a high incidence of associated complications which often require surgical intervention. Indeed, it has been estimated that, largely because of these complications, 50% of all diabetic patients will require surgery at some time during their lives (1).

The disease diabetes mellitus is considered to increase perioperative risk. These conclusions are based on large retrospective studies without matched patient controls (2, 3). Recently other but smaller retrospective studies in well-run clinics have indicated that, when matched for operative procedure, cardiovascular disease, sex, age and weight, there was no significant difference in mortality or morbidity in diabetic patients when compared to non-diabetic patient groups (4, 5). Although it should be added that this observation does not apply to diabetic patients undergoing open heart surgery (6). Thus, it would appear that the disease diabetes mellitus itself does not necessarily increase perioperative morbidity and mortality; the end organ complications of diabetes determine the risk factor.

The overall goal in the management of the diabetic surgical patient should be to ensure that the morbidity or mortality does not exceed that found in a similar non-diabetic population. This will necessitate careful evaluation of the complications of diabetes, especially the late vascular complications, as well as the status of the glycaemic and metabolic control.

As diabetes is considered to represent at least two disease processes, which may require different perioperative management; the currently used classification will be presented.

CLASSIFICATION OF DIABETES

A new classification has recently become established (7); two main types are described in idiopathically occurring diabetes:

Type I, insulin-dependent diabetes mellitus (IDDM) which was formerly known as juvenile onset diabetes but can occur at any age. The disease may be unstable (brittle diabetes) and glycaemic control difficult. Insulin is mandatory to prevent ketosis and maintain life. Management is with subcutaneously administered insulin once to four times daily but recently a continuous subcutaneous infusion is being popularized. This latter technique must be combined with frequent home monitoring of blood glucose, (preferably using a reflectance meter) to achieve "tight control" as well as careful attention to diet. It is known as the open-loop technique in contrast to the closed-loop method (the artificial pancreas) where the data from a continuous blood glucose monitor is computerized and controls the rate of an insulin infusion. Although this technique has been effectively used in open heart surgery it needs close supervision and is complex and expensive (6).

Type II, non-insulin-dependent diabetes mellitus (NIDDM) was previously called maturity onset diabetes but can also occur at any time during life. This disease manifests itself in both the obsese and non-obese population. There is peripheral insulin resistance and ketosis may occur during severe stress. Type II patients are usually treated by diet alone or by diet and oral hypoglycaemic drugs. However, if glycaemic control is poor, due for instance to the transient stress of illness or surgery, insulin therapy is advisable. When intermittent insulin therapy is considered it is important to exclusively use very pure insulins of the modern human type in order to reduce the risk of sensitisation.

Finally, other types of diabetes are described which are associated with various hormonal diseases, the effect of drugs or gestation.

PREOPERATIVE EVALUATION

This should include an assessment of the glycaemic and metabolic control; cardiovascular status and assessment of diabetic neuropathy and nephropathy if present.

Much of the evaluation may be done during the visit to the preanaesthetic clinic in consultation with the endocrinologist and save hospitalization time. Nevertheless it is still advisable to admit the patient 2 or 3 days preoperatively in order to permit further studies and optimize diabetic control if required.

ASSESSMENT OF BLOOD GLUCOSE AND METABOLIC STATUS

Glycohaemoglobin (HbA$_{1c}$). The adequacy of blood glucose control in both Type I and II diabetics over the previous few weeks may be guaged by measurement of the glycohaemoglobin level; this is normally 3-6% of the total haemoglobin but values over 11% indicates persistantly poor control regardless of what an isolated blood or urine glucose measurement reveal (8). It takes one to four days to get the results of this test so that it should be done during the preanaesthetic visit in order to provide management guidelines before surgery.

Urinary glucose. Determination of the urinary glucose as a basis for insulin therapy is of little value in the surgical patient. Not only is the test retrospective but the renal threshold for glucose, which has a large inter-subject variability, can also alter during the stress of illness and surgery (9). However, a routine preoperative check for ketonuria should be done.

Preoperative blood glucose monitoring. If circumstances permit blood glucose should be measured several times before surgery especially if no HbA$_{1c}$ level is available. Instability or hyperglycaemia and ketonuria as well as an elevated HbA$_{1c}$ will necessitate a change to multiple injections of a short acting insulin or an intravenous insulin infusion if rapid control is required.

Metabolic status. Base excess, plasma potassium, chloride, urea and creatinine determinations should be done to assess metabolic homeostasis. Hypokalaemia is not unusual in diabetic patients receiving diuretic therapy for congestive cardiac failure or hypertension. Reversible deterioration of hyperglycaemia sometimes occurs in NIDDM due to hypokalaemia or intracellular potassium depletion (10). Potassium abnormalities must be corrected preoperatively since they predispose to cardiac arrhythmia during anaesthesia.

ASSESSMENT OF CARDIOVASCULAR STATUS

A recent survey of deaths in 448 medical diabetic patients under 50 years of age showed that cardiovascular disease was the major cause of death (11). Similarly it is the cardiovascular status of the diabetic surgical patient which determines the anaesthetic risk (2, 8).

Coronary artery disease occurs 3-4 times more frequently in the diabetic population than in an age-matched non-diabetic group (8, 12). Also when diabetic patients, especially obese females, suffer a myocardial infarction there is a higher mortality rate than in non-diabetic subjects (12). This may happen because there is more extensive but less overt atherosclerotic disease affecting the smaller coronary arteries in Type I diabetes, or an increased incidence of arrhythmia in Type II patients (13). A specific diabetic cardiomyopathy may develop impairing left ventricular function (12, 14). Futhermore, sudden cardio respiratory arrest may occur in patients with diabetic autonomic neuropathy (12, 15). This complication may also account for the pain-free or silent myocardial infarction which is sometimes encountered in the diabetic population. Atherosclerosis is a frequent complication of diabetes and can result in systolic hypertension.

All diabetic patients should have a careful preoperative cardiovascular assessment which should include a 12 channel ECG, electrolyte determination and blood pressure measurements, done both whilst standing and lying down. Diabetic autonomic neuropathy can result in hypotension whilst standing yet hypertension in the supine position (16). Cardiac pathology, if present, should be evaluated in consultation with a cardiologist and cardiac function optimized by introducing or adjusting cardiac medication.

PREOPERATIVE CARDIAC MEDICATION MAINTENANCE OR MODIFICATION

Beta adrenergic blocking agents. These have a slight hyperglycaemic action but the real concern is that theoretically they may mask the symptoms of hypoglycaemia. However, a clinical investigation found that impending hypoglycaemia could still be discerned by Type I patients taking beta blockers and that over a period of 8 months they were no more prone to hypoglycaemia or hypoglycaemic unconsciousness than matched diabetic controls (17). Although $beta_2$ receptors are involved in the release of insulin, it appears that this mechanism is not seriously affected in NIDDM patients taking non-selective betablockers (18). A study in IDDM patients showed the neither propranolol (non-selective) nor metoprolol ($beta_1$-selective) potentiated the glucose-lowering effect of insulin. In contrast, blood glucose recovery after insulin was significantly reduced by propranolol but not by metoprolol (19).

Furthermore, during hypoglycaemia, propranolol caused severe bradycardia and an elavated diastolic blood pressure whilst recovery of the free fatty acid level was inhibited; these effects were milder with metoprolol (19). If diabetic cardiac patients are taking non-selective beta blockade we modify the therapy to a cardio-selective $beta_1$-blocker before surgery. We also continue this therapy into the operative day and give standard premedication (9).

Calcium antagonists. Nifedipine induces glucose intolerance in non-diabetics and exacerbates that in diabetic patients. Blood glucose should be regularly monitored in diabetic cardiac patients taking this drug (20). In contrast, verapamil improves glucose intolerance in NIDDM patients (21). At present, however, the general consensus is that calcium antagonists do not seriously disturb glucose metabolism (22). We continue therapy of these drugs into the surgical day.

Diuretics. The thiazide diuretics are mildy diabetogenic and are best avoided in diabetic patients with cardiovascular disease. Furosemide does not have this effect but hypokalaemia can develop which is particularly dangerous in these patients during anaesthesia.

Antihypertensive agents. Drugs like methyldopa, prazozine and clonidine tend to cause a fall of blood pressure whilst in the upright posture. They are not advisable in patients with diabetic autonomic neuropathy since orthostatic hypotension may be exacerbated (22). We are reluctant to continue specific antihypertensive therapy into the preoperative period in diabetic patients with cardiovascular disease who may also have overt autonomic neuropathy.

Catopril. No untoward effect on blood glucose control has been recorded. It appears to be a suitable drug in the management of hypertension in diabetes mellitus as it appears to have little effect on postural blood pressure control (22).

SURGICAL STRESS AND THE DIABETIC SURGICAL PATIENT

Surgical procedures can cause marked metabolic changes even in healthy patients and in diabetic patients can seriously complicate the control of the blood glucose and metabolic homeostasis. During stress raised plasma levels of cortisol, catecholamines and glucagon both inhibit the action of any insulin present and also mobilize substrates especially glucose and free fatty acids. The diabetic cardiac patient is then particularly at risk for glucose, which is the main energy source for the ischaemic myocardium, cannot be utilized in the absence of insulin. In addition free fatty acid levels become inappropriately elavated under these catabolic conditions. Free fatty acids are easily metabolized as an energy source by the normal myocardium but in diabetes very high levels may be associated with increased myocardial oxygen consumption and a predisposition to arrhythmia (12, 14). A continuous intravenous infusion of glucose -insulin-potassium is an effective way of providing easily available substrate during stress and protecting against cardiac catastrophe (23). The efficacy of this technique has been demonstrated in diabetic patients following myocardial infarction where the mortality rate was reduced from 42% to 17% (13).

In the presence of cardiac pathology it must be emphasized that, except for small and short surgical procedures in well controlled NIDDM, continuous intravenous insulin therapy is strongly advised.

Diabetic microangiopathy
There should be a check for the late vascular complications in other end organs. Coronary microangiopathy has been mentioned but lesions may develop in the kidneys, the peripheral nerves and in the eyes. Proliferative retinopathy could result in perioperative retinal haemorrhage and it is appropriate to treat this with photocoagulation before major surgery.

DIABETIC NEUROPATHY
Neuropathy develops in both Type I and II diabetic patients. The incidence increases with the duration of the diabetes so that 50% of diabetics will suffer from this lesion after 25 years (24).

Sensory neuropathy
The commonest form of diabetic neuropathy is distal, symmetrical neuropathy characterized by peripheral burning pains and tingling (25). This usually start in the feet and legs; the lesion then ascends to the arms and finally to the trunk and scalp. Sensory neuropathy is often accompanied by motor and/or autonomic neuropathy. Sensory and motor lesions will influence the anaesthesiologists decision on anaesthetic technique. Regional anaesthesia, a favoured technique in diabetic

patients, may not be advisable. The pain threshold may also be lower in sensory neuropathy which will need careful perioperative analgesic appraisal.

Autonomic neuropathy

Measurable signs of autonomic neuropathy occur frequently in diabetic patients. This complication is often overlooked by anaesthesiologists to the detriment of the patient for it is associated with a high mortality rate (26, 27). Sudden death may occur especially if atherosclerotic cardiovascular disease is also present (26). Another unpleasant feature is that cardiorespiratory arrest has been recorded during or immediately after anaesthesia although no evidence of myocardial infarction, cardiac arrhythmia or hypoglycaemia was found at that time; the arrests were considered to be a specific complication of diabetic autonomic neuropathy (15).

Clinically the neuropathic lesions cause a wide variety of symptoms; those of importance in relation to surgery include tachycardia and postural hypotension, abnormal pupillary reactions with loss of the light reflex and gastro-intestinal dysfunction with gastroparesis (25, 27).

Both the cardiac nerves and the sympathetic vasomotor fibres are affected (27). Cardiac vagal impairment occurs first, hence tachycardia is an early sign of involvement; it is followed later and in more advanced cases by sympathetic denervation (28). Measurement of beat to beat heart rate changes during forced breathing is a simple and reliable bedside method of establishing a diagnosis of impaired vagal control (29). Severe impairment of vagal heart rate control is recorded by an inspiration-expiration difference of less than 5 beats per minute (28). The heart rate responses caused by standing are mainly vagally mediated but also depend on intact adrenergically mediated vasoconstriction; a similar lack of heart rate response to standing is encountered in autonomic neuropathy. These two tests, easily performed by the anaesthesiologist, are the best methods of assessing the incidence and severity of parasympathetic and sympathetic impairment of cardiac control (30).

In autonomic cardiac neuropathy the normal variability of the heart rate to intrinsic and extrinsic factors is reduced or even absent; there is an increased risk of cardiac arrhythmia due to autonomic imbalance and the effect of cardioactive drugs may be unpredictable. Patients are particularly sensitive to the vasodilating action of anaesthetic agents since compensatory vasoconstriction may be absent. Yet there may be an increased (denervation) sensitivity to both endogenous or exogenous circulating catecholamines (12, 27). Unheralded cardiorespiratory arrest may happen at any time during or after anaesthesia (15). Pain-free myocardial infarction may occur (8). Certainly these patients deserve and should have optimum observation and monitoring.

Finally diabetic gastroparesis may provide another anaesthetic hazard. Gastric emptying of solids (but not fluids) is markedly delayed with undigested food remaining in the stomach after an overnight fast. Metoclopramide was found to normalize delayed solid food emptying rates (31). As these patients are also susceptible to nausea and vomiting it is wise to include metoclopramide with the premedication.

DIABETIC NEPHROPATHY

This lesion is, after cardiovascular disease, one of the most frequent causes of death in diabetes mellitus (11, 26). Renal complications should be assessed initially by determination of the plasma creatinine, urea and electrolytes (10). A reduced glomerular filtration rate will predispose to fluid retention and electrolyte disturbances. The metabolism and excretion of anaesthetic drugs will be impaired. Nephrosis may develop causing hypoalbuminaemia which will affect the plasma binding of many drugs; subsequent oedema will require high doses of diuretic and then incur electrolyte abnormalities which will predispose to cardiac arrhythmia. Renal failure may prolong the action of insulin for, although it is resorbed by the kidney, it is cleared by renal and hepatic metabolism.

GESTATIONAL DIABETES

Blood glucose control may be tricky in these patients who are prone to hyperglycaemia and ketoacidosis especially during delivery. However, maternal insulin requirements are markedly reduced after birth (8), Again continuous insulin-glucose infusion is strongly advised in the management of gestational diabetics during parturition or during surgery at term (8, 32).

DIABETIC KETOACIDOSIS

Diabetic patients for emergency surgery may present with

ketoacidosis. If this condition is confirmed operation should be delayed 4-5 hours while the patient is given standard therapy for ketoacidosis so that at least partial correction has occurred before surgery (33). This is important because untreated ketoacidosis is associated with a high surgical mortality. The metabolic derangement also causes symptoms which resemble an abdominal emergency and the symptoms may disappear when treated (8, 23).

PREOPERATIVE AND INTRAOPERATIVE GLYCAEMIC CONTROL

Hypoglycaemic drugs

NIDDM patients treated with hypoglycaemic drugs may need to have their therapy modified before surgery.

1. Sulphonylureas stimulate the release of endogenous insulin from the beta cells of the pancreas; they can cause hypoglycaemia. Long-acting sulphonylureas like chlorpropamide should be withdrawn and substituted by shorter acting ones like Glibenclamide or Tolbutamide. Chlorpropamide has a half-life of 36 hours which may extend to 200 hours in renal disease (34). Hypoglycaemic coma has been recorded in the elderly up to 60 hours after administration of the drug (35). In addition, it exerts an antidiuretic action and is contraindicated in cardiac diabetic patients (9).

2. Biguanides are considered to act by promoting the anaerobic metabolism of glucose but the also inhibit hepatic lactate disposal. Lactic acidosis may be precipitated by poor perfusion states or hepatic disease. Biguanides (Phenformin) should be discontinued at least 48 hours before surgery and short-acting sulphonylureas or insulin therapy commenced.

If control is poor in NIDDM patients or if anything more than minor surgery is planned it is advisable to use an intravenous insulin infusion intraoperatively.

Insulin therapy

1. No intraoperative insulin or glucose. Some anaesthesiologists still cling to the apparent success of the management proposed over two decades ago where insulin and glucose is omitted on the day of surgery (36). This facilitates the task of the anesthesiologist, who avoids

complicated and potentially dangerous insulin regimes but comprimizes the patient, who is obliged to respond with an inappropriately high catabolic response which will increase postoperative morbidity.

2. Subcutaneous insulin bolus or intravenous bolus therapy. Subcutaneous insulin on the morning of surgery has a depot effect which must be covered by intravenous glucose. Furthermore absorption is unreliable during poor peripheral perfusion which may occur during surgery due to stress, shock or hypothermia. It has been shown that arbitrary insulin regimens, which preoperatively recommend 1/3 - 1/2 of the normal daily insulin requirements given subcutaneously, fall short of their intended goals (37,45).

Intermittent intravenous insulin bolus therapy titrated in relation to blood glucose levels has been recommended (37). But insulin has a plasma half-life of 9 minutes (34). In addition, insulin receptors are saturated and exert maximal affect at moderate levels of circulating insulin so that a small, continuously administered dose will be more efficient and effective than intermittant or large bolus doses.

3. Continuous infusion of insulin A continuous subcutaneous insulin infusion (0,5 units insulin/hour) given by a portable pump has achieved satisfactory glycaemic control during minor surgery under general anaesthesia (38). However, this is not an appropriate method of administration during major surgery.

Most modern protocols agree that an intravenous infusion of insulin is the most suitable method of peroperative administration during all types of surgery (6, 23, 32).

An independent intravenous insulin infusion (0,5-2 units/hours) given by syringe pump is commonly employed. The rate is adjusted manually according to frequent blood glucose determinations. This open-loop technique has been used successfully when there is ketoacidosis or hyperglycaemia with insulin resistance.

A recent study using this method reported good control during open heart surgery where insulin requirements tend to be higher than for other surgical procedures and severe metabolic disturbances may develop. Excellent control also has been achieved during this type of surgery using the "artificial pancreas" or closed-loop system (39).

A combined insulin and glucose infusion has been recommended (23, 40). We prefer this method because we feel it is safer; if the substrate infusion stops, so does the insulin which only has a short half-life. Adsorption of insulin on glass or plastic may reduce the available insulin but discarding the first 25-50 ml of solution or adding several ml of the patients' own blood will circumvent this problem (10, 40).

Classic or arbitrary glycaemic control regimes

1. Avoid hypoglycaemia: blood glucose level below 3 mmol/litre (55 mg/dl)
2. Avoid ketoacidosis
3. Avoid hyperosmolar states: blood glucose level above 33 mmol/litre (600 mg/dl). Hyperglycaemic hyperosmolar non-ketotic coma manifests itself above a blood glucose of 33 mmol/litre and a plasma osmolality greater than 320 milliosmoles (41).

   These arbitrary regimens, which often use subcutaneous insulin dosage not commensurate with the metabolic or surgical stress, do little to prevent postoperative metabolic derangement and excessive catabolism.

Tight control regimens

Many physicians now consider that the long-term maintanance of the blood glucose at "normal levels" (4.5-6.0 mmol/litre or 80-110 mg/dl) will prevent or reduce the incidence and severity of diabetic end organ complications. Some success has been achieved in neuropathic and nephropathic lesions but other results are conflicting and the long term effects are unknown (42, 43).

There are no studies to date which support tight control of blood glucose during surgery. However, it is generally believed that good perioperative control is beneficial and that it reduces the risk of postoperative infection, improves conditions for wound healing and promotes better haemostatic regulation. No "normal" blood glucose concentrations during surgery in diabetics have yet been formulated but the tighter the control the more frequent the blood glucose should be measured. In those clinics where rapid determinations are not easily available we recommend the use of strips (Dextrostix) and a reflectance meter (9). During surgery hourly measurements suffice but should be done more frequently (15-30 minutes) during rapid changes or near safe limits.

Reflectance meters: These monitors are small, portable and cheap and should be available in every OR complex or IC unit. Clinical assessments, both during OR and home use, showed that they were reliable, gave a good correlation with standard glucose measurements and provided satisfactory guidance for blood glucose control (44, 45).

Our clinic does not use very tight control but comprimizes, and sets intraoperative blood glucose limits between 5.5-15.0 mmol/litre (100-270 mg/dl).

PRE- AND INTRAOPERATIVE MANAGEMENT IDDM

1. Admission 48 hours presurgery
   -glycaemic control reassessed
   -cardiovascular, neurological and renal status reviewed
   -biochemical measurements (and glycohaemoglobin)
2. Unstable or brittle diabetics -- soluble insulin control
3. No subcutaneous insulin on day of surgery
4. 6.00 AM day of surgery, 500 ml 5% glucose infusion commenced containing one quarter daily soluble insulin requirements, infusion rate 80 ml/hour. Blood glucose measured.
5. If patient also has been maintained on lente insulin, equivalent soluble insulin requirement is estimated:
   Daily lente insulin units x 1.5 = extra soluble insulin units.
6. Standard premedication. Antianginal therapy in cardiac patients maintained (cardioselective beta blockers, calcium antagonists and nitrates).
7. Blood glucose monitored on arrival in OR (8.00 AM) but if later on schedule blood glucose monitored at least every 2 hours presurgery.
8. Blood glucose in OR < 5.5 mmol/litre (100 mg/dl) glucose/insulin infusion stopped and 5% glucose only given. If 3 mmol/litre (55 mg/dl) or less --> 15 ml 50% glucose i.v.
9. Blood glucose > 15 mmol/litre (270 mg/dl) 5 units soluble insulin added to infusion.
10. Intraoperatively glucose/insulin infusion 80 ml/hour always as independent infusion from blood or IV fluids. No additional glucose or lactate containing infusion.
11. Blood glucose measured hourly during operation as well as plasma potassium and base excess. More frequent measurements if rapid changes or near lower "safe" limit.
12. Persistent blood glucose > 15 mmol/ litre --> soluble insulin infusion (1-5 units/hour) by syringe pump; 30 minute blood glucose

measurements.

PRE AND INTRAOPERATIVE MANAGEMENT NIDDM

1. Admission 24-48 hours pre surgery
   -glycaemic control reassessed
   -cardiovascular, neurological and renal status reviewed
   -biochemical measurements
2. Surgery postponed 48 hours in patients still on biguanides
3. Soluble insulin commenced if poor glycaemic control
4. No sulphonylurea on day of surgery
5. 6.00 AM day of surgery 500 ml 5% glucose with 4-6 units soluble insulin commenced rate 80 ml/hour. This insulin dose is decided on the preoperative adequacy of diabetic control. Blood glucose measured.
6. Patients recently on a long-acting sulphonylarea (chlorpropamide) not given insulin until first blood glucose measurement available.
7. Standard premedication, antianginal therapy maintained in cardiac diabetics.
8. Subsequent intraoperative management as for IDDM.

14

1. Root HF: Preoperative care of the diabetic patient. Post Grad Med 40: 439–444, 1966.
2. Galloway JA, Shuman CR: Diabetes and surgery: a study of 667 cases. Am J Med 34: 177–191, 1963.
3. Kahn O, Wagner W, Bessman AN: Mortality of diabetic patients treated surgically for lower limb infection and/or gangrene. Diabetes 23: 287–292, 1974.
4. Walsh DB, Eckhauser FE, Ramsburgh SR, Burney RB: Risk associated with diabetes mellitus in patients undergoing gall bladder surgery. Surgery 91: 254–257, 1982.
5. Hjortrup A, Sørensen C, Dyremose E, Hjortsø NC, Kehlet H: Influence of diabetes on operative risk. Br J Surg 72: 783–785, 1985.
6. Elliott MJ, Gill GV, Home PD, Noy GA, Holden MP, Alberti KGMM: A comparison of two regimens for the management of diabetes during open heart surgery. Anesthesiology 60: 364–368, 1984.
7. National Diabetes Data Group: Classification and diagnosis of diabetes mellitus and other categories of glucose intolerance. Diabetes 28: 1034–1057, 1979.
8. Reynolds C: Management of the diabetic surgical patient. A systemic but flexible plan in the key. Post Med 77: 265–279, 1985.
9. De Lange S: Management of the diabetic patient - preoperative, intraoperative (during bypass) postoperative. In: Stanley TH, Petty WC (eds), Anesthesia and the cardiovascular system. Martinus Nijhof Publishers, Boston pp 29–36, 1983.
10. Podolsky S: Management of diabetes in the surgical patient. Med Clin North Am 66: 1361–1372, 1982.
11. Tunbridge WMG: Factors contributing to deaths in diabetics under fifty years of age. Lancet 2: 569–572, 1981.
12. Opie LH, Tansy MJ, Kennelly BM: The heart in diabetes mellitus. Part II. Acute myocardial infarction and diabetes. S Afr Med J: 256–261, 1979.
13. Clark RS, English M, McNeill GP, Newton RW: Effect of intravenous infusion of insulin in diabetics with acute myocardial infarction. Br Med J 291: 303–305, 1985.
14. Shapiro M: A prospective study of heart disease in diabetes mellitus. Q J Med 53: 55–68, 1984.
15. Page MMcB, Watkins PJ: Cardiorespiratory arrest and diabetic

autonomic neuropathy. Lancet 1: 14-16, 1978.

16. Olshan AR, O'Connor DT, Cohen IM, Mitas JA, Stone RA: Baroreflex dysfunction in patients with adult-onset diabetes and hypertension. Am J Med 74: 233-242, 1983.

17. Barnett AH, Leslie D, Watkins PJ: Can insulin-treated diabetics be given beta-adrenergic blocking drugs? Br Med J 280: 976-978, 1980.

18. Groop L, Tötterman KJ, Harno K, Gordin A: Influence of betablocking drugs on glucose metabolism in patients iwth non-insulin dependent diabetes mellitus. Acta Med Scand 211: 7-12, 1982.

19. Lager I, Blohme G, Smith U. Effect of cardioselective and non-selective beta-blockade on the hypoglycaemic response in insulin-dependent diabetics. Lancet i: 456-462, 1979.

20. Charles S, Ketelslegers JM, Buysschaert M, Lambert AE: Hyperglycaemic effect of nifedipine. Br Med J 283: 19-20, 1981.

21. Rödjmark S, Anderson DEH: Influence of verapamil on glucose tolerance. Acta Med Scand S 681: 37-42, 1984.

22. Eppinga P, Leemhuis MP: De behandeling van hypertensie bij patienten met diabetis mellitus. Ned Tijdschr Geneeskd 129: 2195-2199, 1985.

23. Alberti KGMM, Gill GV, Elliot MJ: Insulin delivery during surgery in the diabetic patient. Diabetes Care 5 (suppl 1): 65-77, 1982.

24. Pirart J: Diabetes mellitus and its degenerative complications: a prospective study of 4400 patients observed between 1947-1973. Diabetes Care 1: 168-188, 252-263, 1978.

25. Thomas PK, Eliason SG: Diabetic neuropathy. In: Dyck, PJ, Thomas PK, Lambert EH, Bunge R (eds). Peripheral neuropathy. 2nd edition. Saunders, Philadelphia, pp 1773-1810, 1984.

26. Teutsch SM, Herman WH, Dwyer DM, Lane JM: Mortality among diabetic patients using continuous subcutaneous insulin-infusion pumps. N Engl J Med 310: 361-368, 1984.

27. Hilsted J: Pathophysiology in diabetic autonomic neuropathy: cardiovascular, hormonal, and metabolic studies. Diabetes 31: 730-737, 1982.

28. Wieling W, Borst C, Van Dongen Torman MA, Van Der Hofsted JW, Van Brederode JFM, Endert E, Dunning AJ: Relationship between impaired parasympathetic and sympathetic cardiovascular control in diabetes mellitus. Diabetolgia 24: 422-427, 1983.

29. MacKay JD, Page MMcB, Cambridge J, Watkins PJ: Diabetic autonomic

neuropathy: the diagnostic value of heart rate monitoring. Diabetologia 18: 471-478, 1980.

30. Wieling W, Borst C, van Lieshout JJ, Sprangers RIH, Karemaker JM, van Brederode JFM, van Montfrans GA, Dunning AJ: Assessment of methods to estimate impairment of vagal and sympathetic innervation of the heart in diabetic autonomic neuropathy. Neth J Med 28: 383-392, 1985.

31. Wright RA, Clemente R, Wathen R: Diabetic gastroparesis: an abnormality of gastric emptying of solids. Am J Med Sci 289: 240-242, 1985.

32. Bowen DJ, Daykin AP, Nancekievill ML, Norman J: Insulin-dependent diabetic patients during surgery and labour. Use of continuous intravenous insulin-glucose-potassium infusion. Anaesthesia 39: 407-411, 1984.

33. Johnston DG, Alberti KGMM: Diabetic emergencies: practical aspects of the management of diabetic ketoacidosis and diabetes during surgery. Clin Endocrinol Metab 9: 437-460, 1980.

34. Larner J, Hayner RC: Insulin and oral hypoglycaemic drugs; glucagon. In: Goodman LS, Gilman (eds), The Pharmacological Basis of Therapeutics. Fifth edition, Maxmillan Publ Co, New York, 1975.

35. Schen RJ, Khazzam AS: Postoperative hypoglycaemic coma associated with chlorpropamide. Br J Anaesth 47: 899-900, 1975.

36. Fletcher J, Langham MJS, Kellock TD: Effect of surgery on blood sugar levels in diabetes mellitus. Lancet 2: 52-54, 1965.

37. Walts LF, Miller J, Davidson MB, Brown J: Perioperative management of diabetes mellitus. Anesthesiology 55: 104-109, 1981.

38. Barnett AH, Robinson MH, Harrison JH, Watkins PJ: Minipump method of diabetic control during minor surgery under general anaesthesia. Br Med J 280: 78-79, 1980.

39. Watson BG, Elliot MJ, Pay DA, Williamson M: Diabetes mellitus and open heart surgery. A simple, practical closed-loop insulin infusion system for blood glucose control. Anaesthesia 41: 250-257, 1986.

40. Alberti KGMM, Thomas DJB: The management of diabetes during surgery. Br J Anaesth 51: 693-710, 1979.

41. Fulop M, Tannenbaum H, Dreyer N: Ketotic hyperosmolar coma. Lancet ii: 635-639, 1973.

42. Boulton AJM, Drury J, Clarke B, Ward JD: Continuous subcutaneous insulin infusion in the management of painful diabetic neuropathy.

Diabetes Care 5: 386-390, 1982.

43. The Kroc Collaborative Study Group: Blood glucose control and the evolution of diabetic retinopathy and albuminuria. A preliminary multicenter trial. N Engl J Med 311: 365-372, 1984.

44. Webb DJ, Lovesay JM, Ellis A, Knight AH: Blood glucose monitors: a laboratory and patient assessment. Br Med J 280: 362-364, 1980.

45. Madsbad S, Adelhøj B, Bigler D, Hilsted J: Evaluation of two methods of rapid blood-glucose monitoring by unskilled personnel during surgery. Acta Anaesthesiol Scand 28: 649-651, 1984.

WHAT ARE MINIMUM MONITORING REQUIREMENTS AND WHAT DO ECHOCARDIOGRAPHY,
EEG'S, AND OXIMETRY OFFER US?

M. F. ROIZEN

WHAT ARE MINIMUM MONITORING REQUIREMENTS?
  The rationale for monitoring is to:
  1. Spot changes before they cause morbidity.
  2. Ensure no harm comes to the patient.
  3. Keep the anesthesiologist alert.
  4. Ensure machines you are using function.

HOW CURRENT TECHNIQUES FIT INTO THESE:
  Rationales will be discussed, especially stressing how
echocardiography, EEG, and pulse oximetry apply.

TRANSESOPHAGEAL ECHOCARDIOGRAPHY (Ref. 1-12)
  Transesophageal echocardiography is a well-established experimental
technique that is being used at about ten medical centers throughout the
world for diagnosing acute intraoperative cardiac events. With this
technique, regional myocardial ischemia and changes in preload, afterload,
and contractility during surgery can be determined with accuracy. In
addition, structural cardiac defects, both preexisting and acute, can
be detected. Transesophageal echocardiography may soon become part of
standard intraoperative monitoring in selected high-risk patients, helping
to decrease morbidity and increase survival. Monitoring with pulmonary
artery catheters may be supplanted by transesophageal echocardiography
in some circumstances, because the latter provides a better estimate of
preload, a prime determinant of cardiac performance. Real-time digital
signal processing may simplify the interpretation of echocardiograms,
making widespread use more practical.

SHOULD ALL PATIENTS UNDERGOING CAROTID ENDARTERECTOMY BE MONITORED WITH
AN EEG?

RATIONALE:
    YES -- Monitoring with an EEG allows detection of cerebral ischemia
before it leads to permanent sequelae, is significantly more specific
and sensitive than other easily usable detection devices, and thus allows
intervention which preserves brain function. (Ref. 13)
    NO -- The incidence of stroke following carotid endarterectomy is
so low and the false positive rate from EEG analysis so relatively high
that clinically significant events would not be decreased and only costs
and anxiety increased.

CONCLUSIONS AND WHAT I DO:
    There is no definitive data to indicate that intervention once EEG
abnormality is present leads to a lower perioperative morbidity, or even
what the sensitivity and specificity of perioperative EEG monitoring is.
We are currently studying this controversy.

PULSE OXIMETRY
    For monitoring to be able to decrease morbidity, it must:
    A. Be useable.
    B. Have a low rate of false positives relative to true positives.
    C. Lead to a treatment that benefits patients.
    D. Not cause harm greater than good.

    At first blush, pulse oximetry fulfills categories A, C, and D,
but its ability to fill category B and its expense are still problematic.
(Ref. 14-15) Its rationale and improvements needed to fit "B" will be
discussed.

REFERENCES:

1. Shine, K.I., Perloff, J.K., Child, J.S., Marshall, R.C., and
    Schelbert, H. Ann Intern Med 92:78-90, 1980.
2. Forrester, J.S., Wyatt, H.L., da Luz, P.L., Tyberg, J.V.,
    Diamond, G.A., and Swan, H.J.C. Circulation 54:64-70, 1976.
3. Pandian, N.G. and Kerber, R.E. Circulation 66:597-602, 1982.
4. Pandian, N.G., Kieso, R.A., Kerber, R.E. Circulation 66:603-611,
    1982.
5. O'Boyle, J.E., Parisi, A.F., Nieminen, M., Kloner, R.A., and Khuri, S.
    Am J Cardiol 51:1732-1738, 1983.
6. Braunwald, E. and Kloner, R.A. Circulation 66:1146-1149, 1982.
7. Horowitz, R.S., Morganroth, J., Parrotto, C., Chen, C.C., Soffer, J.,
    and Pauletto, F.J. Circulation 65:323-329, 1982.
8. Beaupre, P.N., Cahalan, M.K., Kremer, P.F., Lurz, F.W., Schiller, N.B.,
    and Hamilton, W.K. (Abstr) Anesthesiology 59 (suppl 3A):A59, 1983.
9. Roizen, M.F., Alpert, R.A., Beaupre, P.N., et al. (Abstr)
    Anesthesiology 59 (suppl 3A):A163, 1983.
10. Schlüter, M., Langenstein, B.A., Hanrath, P., Kremer, P., and
    Bleifeld, W. Circulation 66:784-789, 1982.
11. Hanrath, P., Schlüter, M., Langenstein, B.A., et al. Br Heart J 49:
    350-358, 1983.
12. Smith, J.S., Cahalan, M.K., Benefiel, D.J., Byrd, B.F., Lurz, F.W.,
    Shapiro, W.A., Roizen, M.F., Bouchard, A., and Schiller, N.B.
    Circulation 72, No. 5, 1015-1021, 1985.
13. Sundt, T.M., Jr., et al. In Advances in Neurology, Vol. 16,
    (Eds. Thompson and Green), Raven Press, New York, 1977, pp.97-119.
14. Kim, J.M. and Mathewson, H.S. Anesthesiology 63:A174, 1985.
15. Fanconi, S., Doherty, P., Edmonds, J.F., Barker, G.A., and Bohn, D.J.
    J Pediatr 107:362-366, 1985.

MANAGEMENT OF ELECTROLYTE ABNORMALITIES

K. C. WONG, M.D., Ph.D.

Introduction

Proper distribution of cations between the intracellular and extracellular space is essential for maintaining homeostasis. Preoperative potassium abnormalities have been of special concern to the anesthesiologist because of its effects on myocardial functions. There is indeed ample evidence to suggest the detrimental effects of hypokalemia and hyperkalemia on myocardial rhythm and contractility, however, there is no good evidence to date to show that anesthetic dysrhythmias are increased in the chronic hypokalemic patient. How can one reconcile such a lack of clinical correlation? The answer is not clear but it is increasingly evident that hypokalemia alone is only one of a large number of factors which influence cardiovascular function during surgery and anesthesia. The complexity of this problem is depicted in figure 1 which shows some of the factors which can produce hypokalemia, and hypokalemia is only one of the contributing factors to cardiovascular instability. Furthermore, other cations such as calcium, sodium and magnesium are very closely coupled to the electrophysiologic functions of potassium. This review will consider some pertinent aspects of electrophysiology which are influenced by changes in concentration of potassium, sodium, calcium and magnesium; and discuss clinical situations during which these cations can influence the anesthetic management of the patient.

Endogenous Cations and Electrophysiology of Cardiac Cell

Proper sodium concentration in the extracellular space is essential for depolarization, the production of action potential of excitable cells, and for its osmotic effect in the extracellular fluid. Calcium sets the threshold of excitation and is also necessary for myocardial contraction. Magnesium is an important cation for a

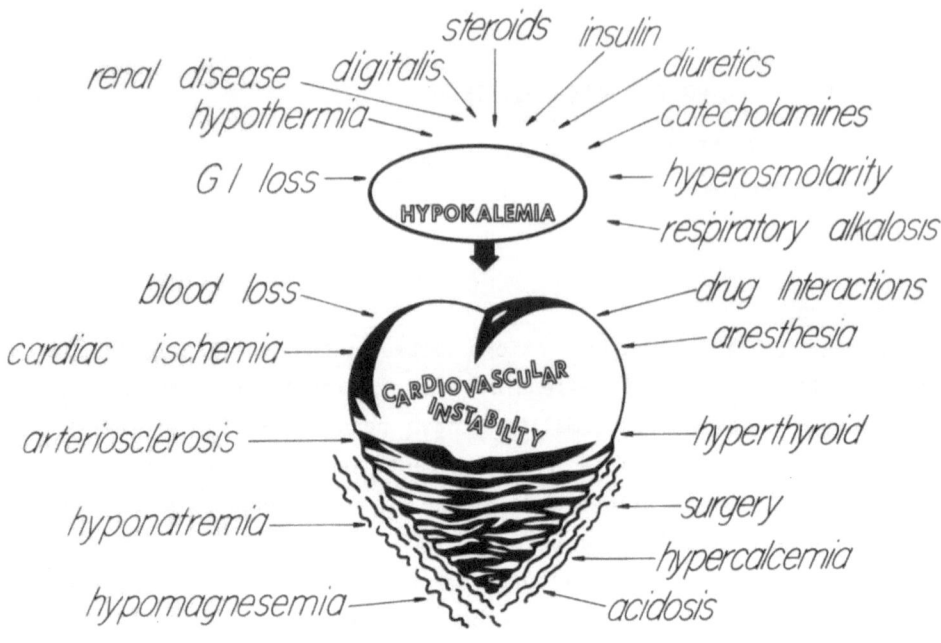

FIGURE 1: Factors contributing to hypokalemia and cardiovascular
instability.

Table. Ionic Concentrations and Potentials in Mammalian Muscle Cells
and Interstitial Fluid*

	Interstitial Fluid	Intracellular Fluid	$E = \dfrac{[ion]_o}{[ion]_i} = \dfrac{60}{Z} \log \dfrac{[ion]_o}{[ion]_i}$ (mv)	
Cations				
N^+	145 um/cm^3	12 um/cm^3	12.1	65
K^+	4 um/cm^3	155 um/cm^3	1/39	-95
H^+	3.8 x 10^{-5} um/cm^3	13 x 10^{-5} um/cm^3	1/3.4	-32
[pH]	[7.43]	[6.9]		
Others	5 um/cm^3			
Anions				
Cl^-	120 um/cm^3	3.8 um/cm^3	31.8	-90
HCO_3	27 um/cm^3	8 um/cm^3	3.4	-32
Others	7 um/cm^3	155 um/cm^3		
Potential	0	-90 mV	31.6	-90

Adapted from Woodbury, 1962.

*o = extracellular; i = intracellular; Z = valence of ion.

variety of cellular functions and has demonstrated to modulate intracellular distribution of calcium. The interrelationship of these cations are depicted in Figure 2.

Potassium is the predominant intracellular cation while sodium is the predominant extracellular cation. The electrolyte solutions of both inside and outside of the cell contain about 155 mEq/L of cations and anions. The ionic distributions and concentration gradients between the intra- and extra-cellular compartments are responsible for generating electrical potentials of mammalian cells for exerting appropriate physiologic functions of the cells. The approximate steady-state ionic concentrations and the electrical potential they generate in mammilian muscle cells and interstitial fluid are shown in Table 1.

The resting membrane potential of about -90 mV, inside with respect to the outside of the cardiac cells, is primarily produced by the transmembrane potassium concentration gradients. Mathematically, the Nernst equation is useful for estimating the resting membrane potential.

$$E = 60 \log_{10} \frac{[K]o}{[K]i}$$

$$E = 60 \log_{10} \frac{4}{155}$$

$$E = -90 \text{ mV}$$

The excitable cell generates an action potential (electrical signal) when its threshold of excitation is reached. The "sodim gate" opens and depolarization occurs by an inrushing of sodim ions through "fast channels", into the cell, thus producing an action potential (Figure 2). The threshold of excitation can be elicited by an electrical, chemical or mechanical stimulus. In the case of the sinoartrial node of the mycardium, there is spontaneous depolarization from influx of calcium through "slow channels" into the cell until the threshold is reached. (Automaticity describes such cells which displays spontaneous depolarization). The resting membrane potential is, therefore, important for governing cardiac excitability and generating an effective action potential. The speed with which action

24

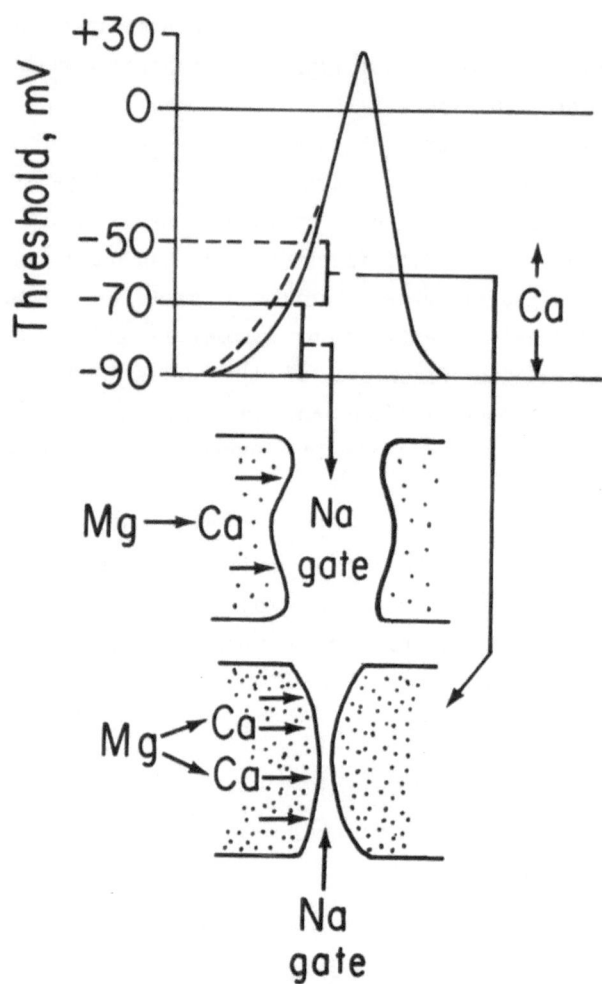

FIGURE 2: The relationship of cations and their influence on action
potentials. Hypercalcemia reduces the rate of sodium influx
and depolarization. Hypocalcemia does the converse.

potential rises determines the velocity of conduction. An increase in the threshold potential (less negative) from e.g. hypercalcium can decrease the rate of sodium influx thus reduce conduction velocity (Figure 2). On the other hand, a reduction in resting membrane potential (more negative) can increase the rate of sodium influx and increase conduction velocity. The complexity of the interaction of cations on electrophysiology is not always simple to provide answers for clinical situations. The action potential of the sinoatrial node is used to illustrate potential effects of potassium abnormalities on electrophysiology and the ECG (Figure 3).

Repolarization of the cardiac cell is also an important function of the transmembrane potassium concentration gradient, since it is the immediate outward movement of K^+ from the cell that repolarizes the cardiac cell. The Na-K pump, then, serves as a physiological "generator" to pump potassium into and sodium ions out of the cardiac cell thus maintaining the proper electrolytic gradients.

Calcium and magnesium are important for controlling cardiac excitability. Calcium sets the threshold of excitation (opening the sodium gate by binding negative sites in the channels for sodium ions). Hypercalcemia elevates the threshold for maximum Na+ permeability while hypocalcemia lowers the threshold. Magnesium may control calcium ion movement and distribution in several types of muscles, thus also regulate cardiac excitability. High extracellular concentrations of magnesium depress atrial ventricular and intraventricular conduction, while hypomagnesemia can produce cardiac arrhythmias including ventricular fibrillation and sudden asystole.

Potassium

Hypokalemia is, by definition, a reduction in serum potassium concentration. Clinically, the only practical means of assessing electrolyte disturbance of the body is by measurement of serum concentrations. However, serum potassium concentration normally only represents 1/39 of intracellular potassium concentration (Table 1). Therefore, it is important to distinguish acute hypokalemia, a reduction of serum potassium concentration, without loss of total body potassium from acute loss of body potassium and chronic loss of potassium.

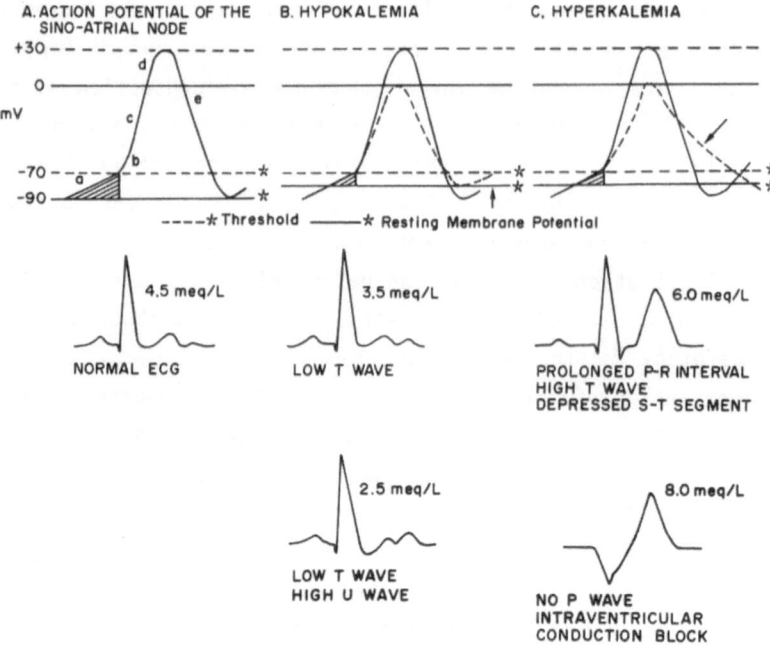

FIGURE 3: Serum potassium abnormality on the electrophysiology of the
sinoatrial node and the ECG.

A. Action potential of normokalemic sinoatrial node
   a. Spontaneous depolarization (influx of Ca^{++} through slow channels)
   b. Threshold potential (open sodium gate)
   c. Maximal rate of depolarization (influx of Na^+ through fast channels)
   d. Overshoot
   e. Repolarization (efflux of K^+ through fast channels)

B. Action potential of chronic hypokalemic sinoatrial node. Intracellular
potassium loss reduces (arrow) the resting membrane potential (more
positive). A smaller action potential is produced. The shaded
triangle area shows that less stimulus is required to excrete the
cardiac cell.

C. Action potential of hyperkalemic sinoatrial node. Hyperkalemia reduces
the resting membrane potential. As the hyperkalemia becomes more
severe, depolarization as well as repolarization are inhibited.

Characteristic ECG changes with corresponding serum potassium changes
are shown below the action potential.

Acute hypokalemia without loss of total body potassium can be induced by transmembrane movement of extracellular potassium ion into cells in exchange for intracellular hydrogen ion as a means of physiologic compensation for acute serum alkalemia. Acute serum acidemia causes shifts of potassium and hydrogen ions in the opposite direction, resulting in an elevation of serum potassium ion concentration. When acid disturbance is chronic, renal mechanisms become more important for maintaining acid/base balance in the body. Acute hypokalemia as a result of transmembrane potassium shift is a common iatrogenic product of hyperventilation during anesthesia and is not a problem in an ASA Class 1 patient. It is estimated that for every 1/10 pH unit increase there could be a 0.5-1.0 mEq/L potassium ion shift into the intracellular compartment. In contrast acute hypokalemia from short term potassium loss such as diarrhea, nasal gastric suction, bowel prep may result in cardiovascular instability. Although there are no hard data to substantiate this clinical impression, a theoretical consideration is that acute losses of potassium from the body has had insufficient time for compensatory mechanisms to take place thus resulting in electrophysiologic disturbances.

Chronic hypokalemia as a result of body loss of potassium over weeks or months can be detrimental to the cardiovascular system. Some causes of chronic potassium loss can be gastrointestinal disturbance, frequent enemas, hyperaldosteronism, digitalis and diuretic therapy. Hypokalemia from digitalis and/or diuretic therapy is the most common type of potassium deficient surgical patient and perhaps is one of the most difficult groups of patients to manage. Indeed these patients usually have significant cardiovascular disease (i.e. cardiac failure, atherosclerosis, hypertension and myocardial ischemic disease). Many chronic hypokalemic patients with serum potassium concentrations below 3 mEq/L do not manifest cardiac arrhythmias except for low T waves on the ECG, suggesting the importance of potassium concentration gradient across the cell membrane for maintaining cardiac stability. On the other hand, the heart of potassium depleted patients is less capable of maintaining homeostasis when challenged by surgery, anesthesia, acid/base imbalance and stress. Animal studies from this laboratory have supported the belief that severe physiologic stress such as asphyxia or catecholamine infusion will increase morbidity and mortality in dogs. On the other hand, the recent publication of Vitez et al suggests that the incidence of intraoperative dysrhythmias are not increased in chronic hypokalemic patients who are asymptomatic during the preoperative phase. In addition to the electrophysiologic disturbance created by the potassium imbalance, intracellular potassium deficit in experimentally induced animals has been associated with poor cardiac contractility and cardiovascular performance. In summary the controversy with regard to the risk of anesthetizing a hypokalemic patient is unresolved. Asymptomatic chronic hypokalemic patients do not seem to carry a higher risk of intraoperative dysrhythmias from other normokalemic patients but this reviewer strongly believes that these patients are less able to compensate for severe physiologic trespass. The clinical impression that acute loss of potassium from the body may be more detrimental to the anesthetized patient is at the present without the support of hard data.

Potassium Therapy

Serum potassium concentration alone is not a reliable reflection of total body $[K^+]$. With the aid of a good history and physical, ECG and objective measurements of potassium loss (e.g. urinary excretion during cardiopulmonary bypass and serum potassium measurements), one can administer potassium more rationally.

The degree of chronic potassium loss, magnitude of contemplated surgery, physical status of the patient and skills of the surgeon and anesthesiologist are all important factors for assessing the surgical risk of the patient. Thus, it is generally agreed that a chronic hypokalemic patient with a serum $[K^+]$ of 3.0 mEq/L is the minimal acceptable level for elective surgery and 3.5 mEq/L is the minimal acceptable level in a digitalized patient.

A 25% reduction of body potassium may exceed 1000 mEq. Theoretically, at least 6-10 days would be required for repletion of such magnitude of potassium deficit based upon a maximal recommended dose of 240 mEq/day and a daily obligatory loss of 50-100 mEq. One cannot expect, then, to replete such deficits by rapid intravenous administration of KCl. In fact rapid IV administration of KCl in experimental animals is rapidly excreted by the kidneys without significant retention of K^+ by the body. However, there are published data to suggest that IV KCl may exert an antiarrhythmic effect in the potassium-depleted patient, especially if the patient is also digitalized. One should be reminded that potassium administration is not inocuous. As many as 1 in 200 patients receiving potassium may suffer a morbid or fatal episode of hyperkalemia. Therefore, there are no absolute rules in deciding rather a hypokalemic patient should be anesthetized or treated. The anesthesiologist must make individualized judgments for a given clinical situation. The readers are reminded of the complex inter-relationship of hypokalemia with other factors which may contribute to cardiovascular instability (Figure 1).

Guidelines for Potassium Administration

1. When time permits, oral potassium 25 mEq every 6-8 hours for one week is the safest and perhaps the most effective way of replenishing body potassium.

2. Intravenous KCl is limited to 0.5 mEq/kg/hr.

3. Do not exceed 240 mEq/24 hr.

4. Monitor the ECG and serum electrolyte.

5. When emergency surgery does not allow at least 12 hours for potassium administration, 0.5 mEq/kg/hr of KCl in 10% dextrose is helpful to facilitate cellular uptake of potassium.

6. Avoid iatrogenic acid-base disturbance.

Acute hyperkalemia is the result of a sudden increase in serum $[K^+]$ and can cause a reduction (more positive) in resting membrane potential with an increase in cardiac excitability. Further increases in serum $[K^+]$ will produce conduction block from poor depolarization and repolarization and finally persistent membrane depolarization and cardiac arrest (Figure 3). An important consideration of acute hyperkalemia during anesthesia is the use of succinylcholine in severely burned, traumatized, cord-injured or myopathic patients. Iatrogenic hyperkalemia from infusion of KCl and stored bank blood are not uncommon. Stored bank blood can release as much as 1 mEq K^+/unit blood/day. The most reliable indices for predicting a dangerous increase in serum potassium following intravenous administration of succinylcholine were shown to be 1) the time elapsed from burn injury to anesthesia and 2) the extent of the burn injury. However, hyperkalemia following injury, and increases in serum potassium to more than 6 mEq/L were observed in patients with total burned surfaces of as little as 8% (i.e. less than the surface of one arm). The K^+-releasing effect begins 5-15 days after injury. It persists for 60-90 days after thermal and crushing injuries, and at least 3-6 months after upper-motor-neuron lesions. There is some question as to whether succinylcholine should ever be used in the presence of chronic, wasting myopathies. Administration of non-depolarizing neuromuscular blocking agent prior to succinylcholine cannot be depended upon to prevent hyperkalemia following succinylcholine in burned patients.

Chronic hyperkalemia implies a gradual increase in extracellular $[K^+]$ with or without a simultaneous increase in intracellular $[K^+]$. This condition commonly exists in chronic renal failure. The fact that these patients generally tolerate serum potassium levels in excess of 6 mEq/L without apparent cardiovascular symptoms supports the importance of an appropriate $[K^+]$ gradient rather than the concentration of K^+ per se across the cell membrane.

Uremic patients needing hemodialysis usually have other concomitant electrolytic disturbances: 1) hyponatremia; 2) hypermagnesemia; 3) hypocalcemia. The major pharmacologic actions of magnesium are vasodilation, central nervous system depression, and neuromuscular blockade. The net effect of these electrolytic disturbances in uremic patients renders them more sensitive to nervous system depressants (i.e. they need less CNS depressants and neuromuscular blocking agents).

Hyperkalemia, however, has the most detrimental effect on myocardial electrical activity (Figure 3). When cardiac function is impaired, treatment of hyperkalemia should include:

1. Monitoring the ECG and serum electrolytes.

2. Intravenous administration of calcium to restore the balance between K^+ and Ca^{++} (as an acute emergency measure by continuous infusion until the sine wave reverts to a normal ECG complex; then rapidly institute other means).

3. Lowering serum K^+
   a. $NaHCO_3$ infusion when hyperkalemia is accompanied by acid-
      osis; the severity of acidosis should be determined by
      blood-gas measurements.
   b. Administration of glucose plus insulin increases cellular
      uptake of K^+; this is given as a 25% solution with 0.5
      unit of regular insulin for each 2 g glucose -- as much
      as 300 ml of glucose may be given in 30 minutes.
   c. Cation exchange resin by mouth or rectum, usually 20-50
      g/day.
   d. Hemodialysis.

Sodium

Sodium imbalance is usually associated with potassium imbalance.
Sodium, in addition to being important for the depolarization of
excitable cells, is also important for its osmotic effect in the
extracellular fluid.

Hyponatremia, in the presence of a decreased extracellular fluid
volume, is encountered when body fluids containing electrolytes which
are lost are replaced with electrolyte-free solutions. Hyponatremia
accompanied by an increased decompensation, in hepatic cirrhosis with
ascites, or in the nephrotic syndrome. Restriction of sodium intake,
while allowing a free fluid intake, contributes to the problem of
hyponatremia with edema. The condition of these patients is
frequently refractory to diuretics until electrolyte balance has been
restored. Poor cardiac performance and increased sensitivity to
nondepolarizing neuromuscular blocking agents are to be expected in
these patients. A serious intraoperative complication is dilutional
hyponatremia secondary to absorption of irrigating fluid during
transurethral resection.

The symptoms of dilutional hyponatremia include:

1. With regional anesthesia, restlessness is an early symptom
and may be associated with irritability and confusion. A serum $[Na^+]$
of 120 mEq/L appears to be borderline between mild and severe
reactions.

2. Hypotension and tachycardia.

3.   ECG changes characterized by widening of the QRS complex and ST segment elevation when [Na$^+$] falls to 115 mEq/L (approx.).

4.   Seizures occur at serum [Na$^+$] 102 mEq/L (approx.).

5.   Ventricular tachycardia or fibrillation may occur at serum [Na$^+$] 100 mEq/L or less.

Principles of treatment of hyponatremia include:

1.   Successful treatment depends upon early detection.

2.   Termination of the surgical procedure and anesthesia usually results in prompt diuresis.

3.   When cardiovascular embarrassment exists, the administration of sodium chloride (NaCl), diuretics and vasoactive agents may be helpful.

4.   Serial monitoring and serum electrolytes.

Recent data suggest that excessive absorption of glycine, the osmotic agent in the TURP irrigating fluid, can produce CNS symptoms to confuse the hyponatremia picture.

Hypernatremia is usually the result of excessive free-water clearance with inadequate intake.   Diabetes insipidus due to head injury is frequently accompanied by hypernatremia and a clouded sensorium.   Chronic steroid therapy is associated with hypernatremia and hypokalemia.

Calcium

Endogenous hyper- and hypocalcemia are usually due to various well known endocrine disorders.   Hypercalcemic nephropathy and hypocalcemic tetany are also well known clinical entities. Hypercalcemia increases the threshold of excitation and hypocalcemia lowers the threshold.   Ionized calcium is the active form and is pH-dependent; thus, alkalosis can reduce serum [Ca^{++}] as well as serum [K$^+$].

The plasma of acid-citrate-dextrose (ACD) blood stored at 4° C has been shown to gain about 1 mEq/L K$^+$/unit blood/day, increased to 32 mEq/L after 21 days of storage.   The pH steadily decreases to approximately 6.5 after 21 days because of cellular metabolism and the formation of lactic and pyruvic acids.   Binding of ionized calcium by the citrate in ACD solution can produce myocardial depression. Hypothermia from rapid administration of cold blood can enhance acidosis and myocardial depression. Thus, hypothermia, acidosis, hypocalcemia and hyperkalemia all can contribute to the syndrome, "citrate intoxication," characterized by hypotension, a narrowed pulse pressure, and elevated left ventricular end-diastolic and central venous pressures. Hepatic disease tends to reduce the metabolism of citrate and enhance its toxicity.

Cardiac contractility is closely dependent upon extracellular calcium concentration. Extracellular calcium is in equilibrium with the mobile fraction of intracellular calcium. Calcium binds the troponin complex in muscle, which normally inhibits cross-bridge formation between actin and myosin, thus producing muscle contraction. The sarcoplasmic reticulum reversibly binds calcium to produce relaxation. Anesthetics (e.g. halothane) can inhibit the positive inotropic effect of calcium. Calcium has been used intraoperatively for its positive inotropic action, but its routine use, prophylactically, for protection against citrate intoxication, although still under consideration, has been generally abandoned.

There are increasing numbers of patients, who have received a calcium channel blocking drug (e.g. verapamil or nifedipine) for cardiac arrhythmias, in need of anesthetic management. Although there are theoretical concerns for the anesthetic management of these patients, clinical experience and published data have not supported the concerns for poor myocardial performance. Patients who are taking calcium channel blockers respond to calcium or other cardiac stimulants. The combined use of verapamil and propranolol can have an additive effect on depression of AV conduction and myocardial contractility.

Magnesium

Magnesium is the second most abundant intracellular cation, having about 1/6 the concentration of potassium. The concentration in plasma is 1.5 to 2.2 mEq/L with about 2/3 as free cation and 1/3 bound to plasma protein. Magnesium is a co-factor for ATP in all its phosphate transfer reactions and is a co-factor for a large number of enzymes. However, it has not received the attention it deserves because the other cations are more conspicuously effected during anesthetic management.

The interaction of magnesium with other endogenous cations on electrophysiology is complex. Magnesium plays an important role in regulating calcium ion movement and distribution in cells, and is frequently overlooked during treatment of cardiac arrhythmias associated with hypokalemia and hypocalcemia. The neuromuscular depressant and vasodilation effects of exogenously administered $MgSO_4$ are better known to the anesthesiologist.

Hypomagnesemia can occur in diarrhea, chronic alcoholism, diabetes mellitus, renal tubular damage, diuretic therapy, and following hemodialysis or cardiopulmonary bypass. The clinical manifestations may include neuromuscular hyperactivity tremor and myoclonic jerks, convulsions and cardiac arrhythmias. The ECG changes associated with magnesium deficit are similar to those seen with hypercalcium. Magnesium deficiency may be associated with hypokalemia and enhanced toxicity to digitalis glycosides. Ventricular tachycardia refractory to potassium, procainamide, lidocaine, diphenylhydantoin and cardiac pacing but responded to $MgSO_4$. Failure to defibrillate in patients following cardiopulmonary bypass was successfully defibrillated with the administration of bolus doses of $MgSO_4$.

Hypermagnesemia is usually due to renal insufficiency, and is manifested by muscle weakness, hypotension, sedation and confusion. The toxemic patient, receiving $MgSO_4$, is another group of hypermagnesemic patients that the anesthesiologist must manage. Deep tendon reflexes are reduced when plasma $[Mg^{++}]$ reaches 4 mEq/L and may be absent at levels approaching 10 mEq/L. At 12-15 mEq/L respiratory paralysis and AV conduction blocks are potential hazards. Intravenous $CaCl_2$ is the effective antagonist of potassium overdose. The neurodepressant effect of Mg^{++} reduces the requirement for depolarizing as well as non-depolarizing neuromuscular blocking agents.

References
1. Aasheim GM: Hyponatremia during transurethral surgery. Canad Anaesth Soc J 20:274-280, 1973.
2. Antman EM, Stone PH, Mueller JE, et al: Calcium channel blocking agents in the treatment of cardiovascular disorders. Part I. Basic and clinical electrophysiologic effects. Annals of Internal Medicine 93:875-885, 1980.
3. Chadda KD, Lichstein E, Gupta P: Hypomagnesemia and refractory cardiac arrhythmias in non-digitaized patient. Am J Cardiol 31: 98-100, 1973.
4. Daniell HW: Arrhythmia in hypokalemia. N Engl J Med 284:1385, 1971.
5. Edmonds CJ, Jasani BM: Total body potassium changes with prolonged diuretic therapy. Am Heart J 85:569-571, 1973.
6. Ellrodt G, Chu CYC, Sing BN: Therapeutic implications of slow channel blockade in cardiocirculatory disorders. Circulation 62: 669-679, 1980.
7. Ghoneim MM, Long JP: The interaction between magnesium and other neuromuscular blocking agents. Anesthesiology 32:23-27, 1970.
8. Giesecke AH, Morris RE, Dalton MD, et al: Of magnesium, muscle relaxants, toxemic parturients, and cats. Anesth Analg 47:689-695, 1968.
9. Gronert G, Theye RA: Pathophysiology of hyperkalemia induced by succinylcholine. Anesthesiology 43:89-99, 1975.
10. Hinkle JE, Cooperman LH: Serum ionized calcium changes following citrated blood transfusion in anesthetized man. Br J Anaesth 43: 1108-1112, 1971.
11. Jasani BM, Edmonds CJ: Kinetics of potassium distribution in man using isotope dilution and whole body counting. Metabolism 20: 1099-1106, 1971.
12. Johnson JE, Hartsuch JM, Zollinger RM, et al: Radiopotassium equilibrium in total body potassium: Studies during ^{43}K and ^{42}K. Metabolism 18:663-668, 1969.
13. Kawamura R, Wong KC, Hodges MR: Intravenous potassium chloride in hypokalemic dogs pretreated with digoxin. Anesth Analg (Cleve) 57:108-113, 1978.
14. Lawson NW, Butler GH, Rat CT: Alkalosis and cardiac arrhythmia. Anesth Analg (Cleve) 52:951-962, 1973.
15. Mazze RI, Escue HM, Houston JB: Hyperkalemia and cardiovascular collapse following administration of succinylcholine to traumatized patient. Anesthesiology 31:540-547, 1969.
16. Miller RD: Complications of massive blood transfusions. Anesthesiiology 39:82-93, 1973.
17. Nayler WG: Calcium exchange in cardiac muscle: A basic mechanism of drug action. Am Heart J 73:379-394, 1967.
18. Price HL: Calcium reverses myocardial depression caused by halothane: Site of action. Am Heart J 73:379-394, 1967.
19. Sack D, Kim ND, Harrison CE Jr: contractility and subcellular calcium metabolism in chronic potassium deficiency. Am J Physiol 226:756-762, 1974.
20. Schernman MM, Sullivan RW, Hyatt KH: Magnesium metabolism in patients undergoing cardiopulmonary bypass. Circulation 39:(Suppl) 235-241, 1969.
21. Scribner BH, Burnell JM: Interpretation of the serum potassium concentration. Metabolism 5:468-479, 1956.

22. Seller RH, Cangiano J, Kim KE, et al: Digitalis toxicity and hypomagnesemia. Am Heart J 79:57-68, 1970.
23. Tobey RE: Paraplegia, succinylcholine and cardiac arrest. Anesthesiology 32:359-364, 1970.
24. Tolmic JD, Joyce TH, Mitchess GD: Succinylcholine danger in the burned patient. Anesthesiology 28:467-470, 1967.
25. Viby-Mogensen J, Hanel HK, Hansen E, et al: Serum cholinesterase activity in burned patients. II. Anesthesia, suxamethonium and hyperkalaemia. Acta Anaesthesiol Scand 19:169-179, 1975.
26. Vitez TS, Soper LE, Wong KC, Soper PG: Chronic hypokalemia and intraoperative dysrhythmias. Anesthesiology 63:130-133, 1985.
27. Wills MR: The Biochemical Consequences of Chronic Renal Failure. Baltimore, University Park Press, 1971.
28. Wong KC, Kawamura R, Hodges MR, et al: Acute intravenous administration of potassium chloride to furosemide pretreated dogs. Canad Anaesth Soc J 24:203-211, 1977.
29. Wong KC, Tseng CK, Puerto BA, et al: Chronic hypokalemia on epinephrine-induced dysrhythmias during halothane, enflurane or methoxyflurane with nitroux oxide anesthesia in dogs. Anaesth Sinica 21:139-146, 1982.
30. Wong KC, Port JD, Steffins J: Cardiovascular responses to asphyxial challenge in chronically hypokalemic dogs. Anesth Analg 62:991-994, 1983.
31. Wang JML, Wong KC, Creel DJ, et al: Effects of glycine on hemodynamic responses and visual evoked potentials in the dog. Anesth Analg 64:1071-1077, 1985.
32. Wright BD, DiGiovanni AJ: Respiratory alkalosis, hypokalemia and repeated ventricular fibrillation associated with mechanical ventilation. Anesth Analg (Cleve) 48:467-473, 1969.

DOES CHOICE OF ANESTHETIC MAKE A DIFFERENCE?

M. F. Roizen

INTRODUCTION

When I accepted this assignment, I felt I could easily defend the position that inhalational anesthetic techniques were most optimal for patients with cardiac disease. I can no longer defend that position for patients with cardiac disease undergoing aortic reconstruction. Today I will present the data that led me to conclude that, prior to 1984, any anesthetic technique could be advocated for patients with cardiac disease, and that it was the anesthesiologist, not the technique, that made a difference in patient outcome. However, recent data imply that choice of agent also plays a role in patient outcome.

DATA PRIOR TO 1984 (Much of this review is taken from Roizen (1) with permission of the author)

The introduction, about a decade ago, of practical techniques for measuring cardiovascular variables (2) coincided with the rediscovery of narcotic anesthesia (3,4) and increased the popularity of performing major vascular and cardiac procedures in very ill patients. These developments naturally led to questioning whether the choice of anesthetic technique (e.g., inhalational versus narcotic) makes a critical difference in outcome in those patients most susceptible to adverse perioperative events (5-9). Anesthetics, narcotic and inhalational, affect the circulation in two ways: (a) directly, as demonstrated in studies on volunteers not undergoing surgery and (b) by modifying the cardiovascular effects of surgery (10). In turn, both actions can be influenced by administration of adjuvant drugs, and by the age, cardiovascular reserve, and disease state of the patient (e.g., chronic heart failure is accompanied by sympathetic stimulation that is depressed by anesthetic agents). Although many reports have discussed the cardiovascular effects of anesthetic agents and five studies prior to 1984 compared outcome after narcotic versus inhalational anesthesia in humans (5-9), controversy still exists as to whether choice of anesthetic agent makes a critical difference to outcome. To answer this question, I reexamined studies in the literature and analyzed them statistically.

The studies considered in this review met the following criteria: they were original studies published after 1964 that reported values for resting, supine subjects; they randomly allocated patients to receive a primarily inhalational or narcotic technique; and they compared the results of these techniques in patients undergoing cardiovascular surgery.

Data from four studies (5-8) met these criteria and were combined with data from another study that did not randomly allocate patients (9). This allowed a statistical approach in which the mean values of each cardiovascular variable from each study provided single data points. Although many other studies met all criteria, only these studies examined cardiovascular effects of one type of anesthetic agent and did not compare that type with another. When data were provided in figures only, they were interpolated to derive mean values and standard deviations. Data were analyzed using analysis of variance with repeated measures, followed by the Student-Newman-Keuls test. Although studies probably varied in reliability, they were accorded equal weight for statistical comparison.

Cardiovascular Effects of Inhalational Agents

Halothane was the only volatile agent used in the comparative studies (5-9). Induction of anesthesia with inhalational agents clearly decreased mean arterial blood pressure and cardiac index. (Isoflurane was not used in the comparative studies and may not affect cardiac index). In patients anesthetized with halothane, surgical stimulation increased heart rate and systemic vascular resistance by numerically small but significant amounts and decreased cardiac index. Noncomparative studies examining the cardiovascular effects of inhalational agents with or without surgery have confirmed these results.

Cardiovascular Effects of Narcotic Agents

Morphine sulfate was the narcotic used in four of the five comparative studies (5-8); fentanyl was the anesthetic used in the fifth study (9). Induction of anesthesia with narcotic agents decreased cardiac index by a numerically small but significant amount. Surgical stimulation significantly increased heart rate, mean arterial blood pressure, and systemic vascular resistance in such patients. The noncomparative studies involving narcotic anesthesia appear to confirm these results, although data for fentanyl varied more among studies than did data on morphine.

Cardiovascular Outcomes for Patients Anesthetized with Inhalational Agents versus Narcotics

Studying patients undergoing open heart surgery, Conahan et al (5) found that 13.1% of patients anesthetized with halothane died, while 15.1% of those anesthetized with morphine died (p > 0.05). Kistner et al (6) reported that changes in the ST segment indicative of ischemia occurred significantly less frequently in patients anesthetized with halothane than in those anesthetized with morphine. In a study by Wilkinson et al (7), 10 of 14 patients (71.4%) given halothane had evidence of myocardial ischemia before bypass, compared with 8 of 12 patients (66.7%) given morphine (p > 0.05). In a study by Moffitt et al (8), 1 of 12 patients anesthetized with halothane as the primary agent produced lactate with sternotomy, compared with 2 of 6 patients anesthetized with morphine (p > 0.5). Thus, in the four randomized studies that examined outcome variables, only one showed a significant difference between narcotic and inhalational anesthetics.

Thus, in 1984, I concluded, as did Conahan and his colleagues in 1973 (5), that no data justify the belief that any narcotic or inhalational agent is superior in its effect on outcome when used for cardiac or vascular anesthesia. The data indicate that skill and care in administration remain more critical to cardiovascular outcome than choice of anesthetic agent. However, within the last two years, data have forced me to change my opinion.

DATA FROM 1984 TO THE PRESENT

Since 1984, I have been greatly influenced by two controlled, randomized studies conducted at the University of California, San Francisco. Although I was disturbed by the data of Reiz et al (11), indicating that isoflurane might worsen myocardial perfusion in areas distal to coronary stenoses, that data has remained controversial and unsubstantiated by outcome data.

In 1985, Smith and coworkers demonstrated that isoflurane plus fentanyl was associated with less intraoperative ischemia than fentanyl alone in high-risk patients (12). At that time, I still believed that perhaps an inhalational anesthetic alone would be even better. But our own study (13) disproved this, and showed that in outcome variables, sufentanil anesthesia alone was associated with less major morbidity than occurred after isoflurane anesthesia alone. These findings occurred in a study of 100 patients randomly assigned to receive one type of anesthesia or the other at the temple of inhalational anesthesia.

CONCLUSIONS

Thus, I am forced to conclude that, given alone, sufentanil is preferable to isoflurane in patients undergoing aortic reconstruction. Because published data indicate that complication rates in aortic reconstruction are as high or higher than our isoflurane group, we postulated that sufentanil is protective. Further study is needed to determine whether all narcotics are protective or whether the combination of sufentanil and isoflurane can produce an outcome as good as, or better than, that found with sufentanil alone.

REFERENCES

1. Roizen, M.F. In Opioids in Anesthesia (Ed. F.G. Estafanous),
    Boston, Butterworth Publishers, 1984, pp. 180-189.
2. Swan, H.J.C., Ganz, W., Forrester, J.S., et al. N Engl J Med
    1283:447-457, 1970.
3. Bailey, P., Gerbode, F., Garlington, L. Arch Surg 76:437-440,
    1958.
4. Lowenstein, E., Hallowell, P., Levine, F.H., et al. N Engl J Med
    281:1389-1393, 1969.
5. Conahan, T.J., Ominsky, A.J., Wollman, H., et al. Anesthesiology
    38:528-535, 1973.
6. Kistner, J.R., Miller, E.D., Lake, C.L., et al. Anesthesiology
    50:324-330, 1979.
7. Wilkinson, P.L., Hamilton, W.K., Moyers, Jr, et al. J Thorac
    Cardiovasc Surg 82:372-382, 1981.
8. Moffitt, E.A., Sethna, D.H., Bussell, J.A., et al. Anesth Analg
    (Cleve) 61:979-985, 1982.
9. Zurick, A.M., Urzua, J., Yared, J.P., et al. Anesth Analg
    (Cleve) 61:521-526, 1982.
10. Roizen, M.F., Horrigan, R.W., Frazer, B.M. Anesthesiology
    54:390-398, 1981.
11. Reiz, S., Balfors, E., Sørensen, M.B., Ariola, S., et al.
    Anesthesiology 59:91-97, 1983.
12. Smith, J.S., Cahalan, M.K., Benefiel, D.J., et al. Anesthesiology
    63:A18, 1985.
13. Benefiel, D.J., Roizen, M.F., Lampe, G.H., et al. Anesthesiology
    (in press).

ANESTHESIA AND THE HYPERTENSIVE PATIENT

E. D. MILLER, JR.

Systemic arterial hypertension is frequently a problem in the
perioperative period. By definition, a blood pressure greater than
160/95 mmHg indicates that a patient has hypertension. However,
hypertension may result from a variety of causes. This presentation
will examine some of the factors involved, the consequences of
hypertension, and the approaches the anesthesiologist might use to
improve patient management during the perioperative period.

PERIOPERATIVE PERIOD

Examination of a potential surgical patient often reveals that
the initial blood pressure is elevated. Since one of the common causes
of preoperative hypertension is anxiety, true preexisting hypertension
seems unlikely because with either sedation or reassurance, blood
pressure returns toward normal levels. However, one should not assume
that these patients will respond to anesthesia and surgery in a normal
manner. Bedford and Feinstein (1) observed that the largest increases
in blood pressure at the time of surgery occurred in a group of patients
who had entered the hospital with elevated mean arterial pressure but
had had a decline in blood pressure by the next morning. In this study,
in twelve patients who had direct arterial monitoring, mean arterial
pressure increased to 152±4 mmHg at the time of intubation. Normotensive
patients and patients with known hypertension preoperatively had
increases of mean arterial pressure to 117±5 mmHg and 129±9 mmHg,
respectively. These patients, who show extreme reactivity to stress,
may be borderline hypertensive patients and are known to have the same
risk factors that true hypertensive patients have (2).

The most common cause of an elevated arterial pressure is preexisting hypertension. Hypertension may be divided into two broad categories: primary or essential hypertension and secondary hypertension.

Secondary hypertension includes hypertension due to identifiable factors, such as primary aldosteronism, stenosis of the renal artery resulting in renovascular hypertension, parenchymal renal disease (eg., nephrosclerosis), and pheochromocytoma. Secondary hypertension comprises about 10% of all patients with hypertension. In most cases, specific treatment of the underlying condition results in complete cure of the hypertension. While these patients represent only a small percentage of all hypertensives, an understanding of their basic pathophysiology may be helpful in the preoperative diagnosis and treatment.

Primary aldosteronism is a condition in which an adenoma in the adrenal gland produces excess amounts of aldosterone. Aldosterone is a potent steroid which causes sodium retention and subsequent potassium excretion by the kidney. With increased sodium retention, effective blood volume is increased and blood pressure becomes elevated. The patient presents with hypertension, hypokalemia, low plasma renin activity, and metabolic alkalosis. Removal of the adenoma results in a cure of the hypertension (3).

Renovascular hypertension occurs when one or both renal arteries become stenotic. In younger individuals, the stenosis is due to fibromuscular thickening of the renal artery, while in older patients, it is due to atherosclerosis. The stenosis causes a decrease in pressure within the kidney, which, in turn, effects the release from the kidney of renin, a protolytic enzyme. Renin acts on a plasma protein to form angiotensin I which is converted to angiotensin II in passage through the pulmonary circulation. Angiotensin II is a potent vasoconstrictor, as well as a stimulus to aldosterone secretion. These two factors work in concert to raise arterial blood pressure. With correction of the stenosis, arterial pressure falls toward control levels if the hypertension has not been too long-standing (4).

Renal parenchymal disease often results in patients with an increased arterial blood pressure. It appears that about 80% of these patients have increased arterial pressure secondary to increased extracellular volume. This increased volume is due to the patient's inability to excrete solutes because of his renal dysfunction. If renal dialysis is employed, blood pressure can be controlled with this therapeutic modality alone. The other 20% of these patients appear to have a renin-dependent hypertension and are greatly helped by inhibition of the renin-angiotensin system (5,6).

Pheochromocytoma still remains one of the anesthetic challenges of today. In the past, operative mortality for removal of this tumor was high. Because of better understanding of the underlying pathophysiology and improvement in drug therapy, this is no longer true. Pheochromocytoma is a catecholamine-producing tumor of neuroectodermal origin that is made up of chromaffin cells. The tumors usually are located within the sympathetic nervous system, and roughly 95% are found in the adrenal medulla. Another 2% of the tumors are located at various sites within the abdomen, and 3% are extra-abdominal.

Hypertension is the clinical hallmark of pheochromocytoma. Fifty percent of the patients have sustained hypertension and many of the other patients have paroxysmal hypertension. Most tumors secrete both norepinephrine and epinephrine, but norepinephrine-secreting tumors predominate. Smaller tumors usually cause more signs and symptoms than do large tumors. Diagnosis is suspected because of signs and symptoms (headache, nervousness, palpations, weight loss, diaphoresis). Rarely, the diagnosis may be made during operation with sudden onset of severe hypertension at time of abdominal exploration. There are several excellent reviews on this subject and the reader is referred to them for more detail (7-9).

PRIMARY HYPERTENSION

While the secondary causes of hypertension are well understood, the common variety of hypertension--essential hypertension--still remains without a specific etiology. Page and McCubbin proposed the mosaic theory of hypertension which linked several factors together. These include heredity, salt intake, psychological influences, and the sympathetic nervous system.

Presently, investigators have begun to look more closely at amounts of catecholamines on target organs, the sodium-potassium transport systems in a variety of cells, and the search for a putative hormone that might initiate or maintain the hypertensive state. Investigators have also sought the nature of a substance called natriuretic factor and have tried to implicate it in hypertension. None of these studies is conclusive. Whether one factor or a combination of factors will be crucial for the development of hypertension remains to be proven (10-12).

Whatever the cause of hypertension, certain hemodynamic findings are similar. First, cardiac output is normal and the hypertension is due to an increased peripheral vascular resistance (13). Second, any stimuli which causes constriction of vascular smooth muscle will have more pronounced effect in the hypertensive patient as compared to the normotensive patient (14). This means that the blood pressure response will be greater in the hypertensive patient at intubation, for example. These exaggerated responses may be modified by appropriate drug therapy.

DRUG THERAPY

In the classic pharmacological study of the importance of drug therapy of hypertension by Freis and coworkers (15), it was well established that the morbidity and mortality of severe hypertension could be greatly decreased if blood pressure was lowered. It appears that the manner in which blood pressure is lowered is not as important as the fact that the blood pressure remains in the normal range. Patients' lack of compliance with drug therapy has been one major reason for the development of new drugs with fewer side effects.

Mild hypertension has been shown to be effectively treated with diuretics. How diuretics lower blood pressure is not known. Patients with essential hypertension have been shown to have a decreased plasma volume. Perhaps diuretics cause the loss of sodium from cells important in blood pressure control.

Beta blockers have been added to the list of drugs which are now used to treat hypertension. Because the antihypertensive effect of such drugs requires weeks for onset, the blockade of β-receptors alone does not adequately explain their mode of action. Beta blockers are known to inhibit renin release, and part of their antihypertensive action may be due to this mechanism.

Much of the drug therapy of moderate-to-severe hypertension has been directed at agents which act directly on the sympathetic nervous system. Guanethidine, reserpine, and prazosin have a predominate effect on the peripheral sympathetic nervous system, while agents such as clonidine and methyldopa work centrally.

Drug therapy aimed at inhibition of the renin-angiotensin system with saralasin and captopril has now been shown to be extremely effective in patients with renovascular hypertension and also, surprisingly, in patients with essential hypertension. Currently, calcium channel blockers which cause relaxation of peripheral vascular smooth muscle may prove to be excellent antihypertensive agents.

Data and experience have now shown that when a hypertensive patient comes to a surgical operation, antihypertensive agents should be continued up to, and after, the surgical procedure. Concern that the sympathetic nervous system dysfunction caused by the antihypertensive agents would result in severe hypotension intraoperatively has not been verified.

In summary, the most important consideration in the care of patients with preoperative hypertension is the recognition that they are hypertensive. This is crucial to their care so that appropriate work-up studies can be done and drug therapy instituted or altered prior to surgery. While severe intraoperative hypertension may be effectively treated, a better course of treatment would be the prevention of such episodes. If the patient is diagnosed as being a hypertensive, appropriate lab work would include BUN, creatinine, serum K+, EKG, and chest x-ray. If history or physical findings suggest cardiac dysfunction, then other tests may be indicated (16). If the patient is presently being treated with drugs, knowledge of the type given and how the drug will be administered postoperatively is necessary. Often, drug therapy is not maximal and may need to be altered during the hospital course.

INTRAOPERATIVE PERIOD

The main intraoperative concern for patients who are hypertensive prior to surgery is protection of the major organs that have potential dysfunction because of the long- standing hypertension. The main organs at risk are the heart, brain, and kidney. Substantial evidence exists that these organs may be severely damaged and that the reserve necessary for adequate function may be lost intraoperatively. For example, cerebral autoregulation is known to be altered (17). Recent data suggest that antihypertensive therapy will partially restore cerebral autoregulation (18). Therefore, the decision whether to use controlled hypotension or to allow blood pressure to decrease significantly for a particular procedure will be based partially on the adequacy of antihypertensive therapy prior to surgery.

Much of the knowledge concerning morbidity and mortality is based on arbitrary limits of blood pressure; so also are the recommendations concerning cancellation of elective surgery (19). A guideline which may be useful is a diastolic pressure greater than 110 mmHg. Then, surgery should be cancelled, and appropriate drug therapy instituted. Since these pressures are seen only in a small minority of patients, surgery need not often be postponed. The majority of patients who are found to have hypertension prior to surgery or who are inadequately controlled have diastolic pressures less than 110 mmHg and can be managed safely intraoperatively (20,21).

The main aim of intraoperative management of the hypertensive patient should be to diminish the large increases in blood pressure often seen at times of intubation, incision, and at completion of surgery. This may be accomplished through the use of potent anesthetic agents or narcotics. Regional anesthesia is also an acceptable form of anesthesia but shows no distinct advantage over general anesthesia. If intraoperative hypertension should occur, treatment with vasodilating agents should be given so that myocardial oxygen demand does not remain high for long periods of time.

It should be appreciated that intraoperative hypertension can occur in normotensive patients as well. Inadequate anesthesia due to vaporizor malfunction or inadequate narcotics results in tachycardia and hypertension. Before beginning treatment with vasoactive agents, the causes of the hypertension must be investigated and corrected. Since carbon dioxide is known to stimulate the sympathetic nervous system, hypercarbia should be eliminated as a potential cause of hypertension (22). Bladder distention, late stages of hypoxia and exogenous administration of catecholamines have all been reported to cause intraoperative hypertension. These latter factors all can cause significant hypertension in normotensive patients. In hypertensive patients, these effects are magnified and have the potential to cause myocardial infarction, stroke, or renal failure.

POSTOPERATIVE PERIOD

In the past decade a great deal of emphasis has been placed on diagnosis and treatment of hypertension for our entire population. Significant decreases in morbidity and mortality have resulted. Anesthesiologists have recognized the importance of blood pressure control preoperatively, and this has influenced the intraoperative management of these patients. Despite these advances, the postoperative treatment of hypertension has been neglected to a large extent. Personal experience has demonstrated more episodes of myocardial infarction and stroke in the immediate postoperative period than at the time of induction. Invariably, the scenario is one of severe hypertension, starting to develop at the very end of surgery, becoming progressively worse in the first few minutes in the recovery room, and leading to acute deterioration of the patient. The problem of hypertension in the recovery room has been appreciated for some time. Gal and Cooperman (23) examined 1844 patients and found that of these patients, 60 had significant elevation of their blood pressure. Sixty percent of these hypertensive patients had a history of hypertension. The major factors responsible for the hypertension were pain (35%), hypercarbia (15%), and emergence excitment (16%). Often the condition was self-limiting but some patients remained hypertensive. It is important to decide whether or not the hypertension seen postoperatively should be treated aggressively. Certainly, the treatment of hypercarbia or pain should be instituted early, and further therapy begun if there is no improvement.

What are the options for treatment of hypertension? Nitroprusside and nitroglycerin have been used frequently to control blood pressure postoperatively. Each drug has its own advantages and disadvantages, but such treatment requires infusion pumps, and in most circumstances, arterial monitoring. Since most recovery rooms are unable to have several patients maintained in this manner, a simpler method is desired. The use of hydralazine and propranolol intravenously greatly simplifies the management of most patients. Hydralazine, 5-10 mg, produces its maximal effect in 10-15 minutes. Similarly, 0.5-1.0 mg of propranolol intravenously potentiates the effects of hydralazine. If it appears that continuous use of hydralazine will be required, long-acting agents such as alpha methyldopa can be started.

Certain surgical operations are harbingers of postoperative hypertension. For example, systemic arterial hypertension necessitating therapy has been reported to occur in 30-60%, or more, of patients undergoing coronary artery bypass surgery (24). Certain factors identify these particular patients, including prior history of hypertension, hypertension on the day prior to surgery, stenosis of the left main coronary artery, and good left ventricular function. The hypertension following coronary artery bypass surgery has been characterized hemodynamically as having an increased systemic vascular resistance and a normal cardiac output (25). The mechanisms responsible for the hypertension seem to be multifactorial and perhaps interrelated. Sympathetic nervous system activity is elevated, as well as activation of the renin-angiotensin system (26). Current studies with the use of MK-422 (a converting enzyme inhibitor) may prove to be beneficial in the prevention of postoperative hypertension (27).

In summary, perioperative hypertension is of concern in the surgical patient. With adequate understanding of the cause of the hypertension, appropriate therapeutic approaches should be used. Such treatment will decrease the demands on the heart and should help protect the brain and kidney from ischemia. A variety of potent vasoactive agents is now available to achieve these aims and should be used when indicated. Through such treatment we should be able to provide better care of the surgical patient at a time of maximum stress.

REFERENCES

1. Bedford, R.F. and Feinstein, B. Anesth. Analg. 59:367-370, 1980.

2. Paul, O. Br. Heart J. 33(supp):116-121, 1971.

3. Gangat, Y., Triner, L., Baer, L. and Puchner, P. Anesthesiology
    45:542-544, 1976.

4. Stanley, J.C., Ernest, C.B. and Fry, W.J. Renovascular
    Hypertension. Philadelphia, W. B. Saunders Company, 1984.

5. Onesti, G., Kim, K.E., Greco, J.A., del Guercio, E.T., Fernandes,
    M. and Swartz, C. Circ Res 36(supp):145-154, 1975.

6. Case, D.B., Atlas, S.A., Sullivan, P.A. and Laragh, J.H.
    Circulation 64:765-771, 1981.

7. Atuk, N.O. Hosp Prac 18:187-202, 1983.

8. Bravo, E.L. and Gifford, R.W. N Engl J Med 311:1298-1303, 1984.

9. Suzukawa, M., Michaels, I.A., Ruzbarsky, J., Kopriva, C.J. and
    Kitahata, L.M. Anesth Analg 62:100-103, 1983.

10. Erne, P., Bolli, P., Burgisser, E. and Buhler, F. N Engl J Med
    310:1084-1088, 1984.

11. Garay, R.P., Elyhozi, J.L., Dagher, G. and Meyer, P. N Engl J Med
    302:769-771, 1980.

12. Plunkett, W.V., Hutchins, P.M., Gruber, K.A. and Buckalew, V.M.
    Hypertension 4:581-589, 1982.

13. London, G.M., Safar, M.E., Sassard, J.E., Lwenson, J.A. and Simon,
    A.C. Hypertension 6:743-754, 1984.

14. Folkow, B., Grimby, G. and Thulesius, O. Acta Physiol Scand
    44:255-261, 1958.

15. Veterans Administration Cooperative Study Group on Antihypertensive
    Agents: I. Effects of treatment on morbidity: Results in
    patients with diastolic blood pressure averaging 115-129 mmHg.
    JAMA 202:1028-1035, 1967.

16. Drayer, J.M., Gardin, J.M. and Weber, M.A. Chest 84:217-221, 1983.

17. Strandgaard, S., Olesen, J., Skinghof, E. and Lassen,N.A. Br Med J
    1:507-509, 1973.

18. Hoffman, W.E., Miletich, D.J. and Albrecht, R.F. Anesthesiology
    58:326-332, 1983.

19. Prys-Roberts, C. Int Anesthesiol Clin 4:18-37, 1980.

20. Goldman, L. and Caldera, D.L. Anesthesiology 50:285-292, 1979.

21. Prys-Roberts, C. Anesthesiology 50:281-284, 1979.

22. Rose, C.E., Althaus, J.A., Miller, E.D. and Carey, R.M. Am J Physiol 245:H924-H929, 1983.

23. Gal, T.J. and Cooperman, L.H. Br J Anaesth 47:70-74, 1975.

24. Roberts, A.J., Niarchos, A.P., Subramanian, V.A., et al. J Thorac Cardiovasc Surg 74:846-859, 1977.

25. Niarchos, A.P., Roberts, A.J., Case, D.B., Gary, W.A. and Laragh, J.H. Am J Cardiol 43:586-593, 1979.

26. Bailey, D., Miller, E.D., Kaplan, J. and Rogers, P. Anesthesiology 42:538-544, 1975.

27. Gomez, H.J., Cirillo, V.J. and Jones, K.H. J Hypertension 1(supp 1):65-70, 1983.

ANESTHESIA FOR CONGENITAL CARDIAC DISEASE

J. ARENS

Some general guidelines can be given for dealing with children with cyanotic heart disease. Specific recommendations will be given for some of the more common syndromes later.

Most patients with cyanotic heart disease should come to the operating room well sedated. One regime is Secobarbital 1 mg/lb; Meperidine 1 mg/lb; Atropine 0.1 mg per 10 lbs. It is important to avoid both bradycardia (cardiac output is often rate dependent) and shunt reversal (e.g. converting a left to right shunt to a right to left one). Increased pulmonary vascular pressures due to straining, crying, over-vigorous ventilation, etc. or decreasing systemic vascular resistance caused by halothane, etc. may produce a right to left shunt with dramatic decreases in PaO_2. Therefore, the patient should ideally remain quiet without straining, coughing or crying during induction. If a tranquil induction cannot be achieved with an inhalation agent, I.M. ketamine (1), though painful, is a useful adjuvant.

Once unconsciousness has been produced, a low dose inhalation or moderate dose narcotic (2) technique with appropriate air/O_2 ratio may be used while a peripheral I.V. is started. It is mandatory that all lines be bubble-free when the patient has an intracardiac defect. An arterial line then is started in an appropriate artery taking into consideration the exact surgical procedure to be done. Succinylcholine 1-2 mg/kg I.V. is given to facilitate endotracheal intubation. If long term postop ventilation is anticipated, nasotracheal intubation is appropriate. A CVP may now be placed, and if either extensive surgery or difficulty in coming off bypass is expected, a second central line may be needed - e.g. one CVP for drip drugs, the other for push drugs. If a persistent left superior vena cava is present, a short left external jugular line may be useful to determine the adequacy of venous drainage from that area. If drainage is inadequate, the left cava may need to be cannulated separately.

If bypass is to be used, prior to bypass the patient's temperature may be allowed to drift since hypothermia during bypass is frequently employed. In order to maintain a reasonable blood pressure and heart rate pancuronium may be used for muscle relaxation. Pancuronium also causes less ganglionic blockade (peripheral pooling) than d-tubocurarine.

Patients with congenital heart defects frequently exhibit very low peripheral resistance once extracorporeal circulation is begun. Mean arterial pressures in the 25-30 mmHg range are common. If the C.I. is high (2.5-3.0 L/m^2/min), urinary output, and other parameters of perfusion are satisfactory, vasopressors generally are not necessary because these patients should have adequate cerebral blood flow. Also, many times pulsatile flow disappears as soon as extracorporeal circulation is instituted. In these cases, unlike patients with coronary artery disease, intervention is not required.

The remainder of bypass is little different from other bypass procedures except when total circulatory arrest is employed. Two other observations are important. First, children with cyanotic heart disease have a greater heparin requirement and 4 mg/k is used initially. Secondly, these patients invariably have metabolic acidosis with a low HCO_3^-.

Coming off the pump requires the team to establish an appropriate Starling Curve for the patient. $CaCl_2$, vasoactive support, volume, etc., are often needed. Appropriate use of pacemakers may also be necessary since heart block may have developed. Reversal of anticoagulation needs to be accomplished with judicious use of protamine.

Transport of the patient to the ICU needs to be done skillfully and expeditiously with transport monitors. In addition, succinylcholine, laryngoscope, styletted tube, and Magill forceps must be immediately available so that reintubation may be promptly performed if accidental extubation occurs.

Bradycardia may occur while opening the sternum. Arrhythmias frequently occur during manipulation of the heart and insertion of cannulae. When the aortic cannula is inserted, the arterial pressure trace needs to be closely observed to detect mechanical obstruction of the aorta by the cannula. Sudden disappearance of the arterial wave form may be due to twisting of the aortic cannula causing subsequent kinking of the aorta. Close communication with the surgeon is obviously a must.

SHUNT OPERATIONS FOR CONGENITAL HEART DISEASE

Some infants with congenital heart disease have too little blood flow going to the pulmonary arteries. In addition, a right to left shunt further decreases the patient's oxygenation. The two most common conditions producing such a scenario are: (a) Tetralogy of Fallot; and (b) transposition of the great vessels with a VSD and pulmonary stenosis.

If the infant begins to deteriorate before a total correction of either of the above can be performed, an operation will be performed to anastomose a portion of the aortic arch or immediate branches to the pulmonary arterial system at a point distal to the pulmonary stenosis (3).

1) Blalock-Taussig - This consists of an anastomosis between the subclavian artery and a pulmonary artery. It is usually performed on the right side, but may be done on either depending upon the anatomy of the aortic arch.

2) The Potts procedure is rarely used any longer but consists of anastomosing the descending aorta to the left pulmonary artery.

3) An operation which has been popularized in the past ten years is the Waterston shunt. This consists of anastomosing the posterior wall of the aorta to the right pulmonary artery (aortic window).

The following three procedures are performed to increase mixing of blood from various chambers.

1) Rashkind - An atrial septostomy is performed with a balloon catheter to increase mixing (e.g. transposition).

2) Blalock-Hanlon - An atrial septostomy is surgically made.

3) Glenn Procedure - The superior vena cava is anastomosed to the right pulmonary artery, and is performed in patients with tricuspid atresia.

If the patient has a pure form of pulmonary stenosis, a <u>Brock</u> procedure may be performed which is a pulmonary valvotomy.

As can be imagined, patients who require such shunts are extremely sick. They are often cyanotic, in right heart failure, hemoconcentrated, with a metabolic acidosis, in poor nutritional condition.

Line placement is always a problem. One must find out which type of shunt is planned and on which side. CVP placement should not be performed on the proposed side for the shunt because an arterial hematoma may make the operation technically difficult if not impossible. Once the subclavian artery is used for a shunt there may be no radial or brachial pulse on that side. Therefore, if an arterial line is planned, it needs to be on the opposite side. The anesthetic technique must protect against increasing a right to left shunt. In general, these cases involve primarily resuscitation. These shunts are often technically difficult and the surgeon may have to push on the heart, etc., causing multiple periods of hypotension. Once the shunt is established, bleeding may be a problem. If the shunt is too large the patient may show pulmonary edema or heart failure. The surgeon may want to measure pulmonary artery pressures directly. If the PA pressure is greater than 2/3 that of the systemic pressure, the shunt is too large and will have to be reduced. Conversely, the shunt may be too small, resulting later in thrombosis. If the shunt is too small persistent hypoxemia, metabolic acidosis, and possibly bradycardia will be noted. If these are noted, revision of the shunt will be necessary.

Children will be allowed to go to 2-4 years of age before being scheduled for definitive surgery if their shunts are working adequately. The larger the child, the less technical difficulty encountered by the anesthesiologist, surgeon and pump technician. Before going on bypass, these shunts must be ligated. Failure to do so results in pulmonary hyperperfusion with the institution of bypass creating surgical problems from massive pulmonary return to the heart.

Remember, positive pressure ventilation post-op will reduce pulmonary blood flow. If the shunt is small, spontaneous ventilation may be better.

PATENT DUCTUS ARTERIOSUS

Today surgical closure of a patent ductus arteriosus (PDA) is most frequently done in neonates with respiratory distress syndrome. The incidence of PDA varies from 15 to 80% depending on birth weight, gestational age, and index of suspicion. Just as a high paO_2 is responsible for closure of a PDA, a previously closed ductus may reopen secondarily to hypoxemia (a new murmur is suddenly noted). Surgical correction is usually dictated by the persistence of respiratory distress or refractory congestive heart failure.

Patients requiring surgery are often very small (less than 2 kilos), intubated, mechanically ventilated, dehydrated and malnourished. In addition, the possibility of necrotizing enterocolitis (NEC) as a complicating feature must be entertained, since the incidence of NEC is higher in neonates with PDA (4). One theory suggests the etiologic cause is desaturated blood reaching the intestine. Another proposes that intestinal blood flow may be impaired secondary to a "diastolic steal" of blood from the intestines to the pulmonary artery (5).

The anesthetic principles for the procedures are basically those of resuscitation. Sufficient FIO_2 is given to maintain a reasonable PaO_2 - e.g. 70-80 mmHg. Line insertion is a challenge. If possible, a right radial A-line is useful to indicate the PaO_2 of arterial blood reaching the brain, especially the retinal arteries. The surgery is usually quite bloodless and is also quick. Fluid replacement and temperature control are as important in these neonates as in any others.

When the ductus is closed, the anesthesiologist should hear the murmur change and/or disappear. In addition, the diastolic pressure rises alone producing a decreased pulse pressure. On occasion, a rise in the systolic pressure will also be noted.

In older children, the closure of the ductus is usually done for one of three reasons:

a) to prevent subacute bacterial endocarditis (SBE) (6)

b) to correct pulmonary hypertension

c) to prevent left or right ventricular failure.

In evaluating these patients perioperatively, it is important to assess:

1) the degree of heart failure.

2) the ratio of pulmonary to systemic blood flow.

3) the degree of pulmonary hypertension.

4) the actual anatomic site of the ductus in relation to the subclavian artery.

It is important to have the A-line placed in the right radial artery in the event that surgical consideration requires clamping of the left subclavian artery during closure. If the clamp should slip off the ductus during the repair, major blood loss can occur. Fortunately, this is rare. Postoperative care is like that provided any thoracotomy.

COARCTATION

Coarctation of the aorta may be associated with other congenital heart defects. However, this discussion deals with the uncomplicated postductal coarctation of the aorta. These children are initially asymptomatic but develop progressive upper body hypertension, and collateral circulation to the organs distal to the constriction. To avoid the complications of hypertension, early surgical correction is urged.

General endotracheal anesthesia with one of the potent inhalational agents is satisfactory. These patients are positioned with the left side up. Bleeding is usually excessive during chest entry because of large collaterals. Once again the arterial line needs to be in the right radial artery since surgical considerations may require clamping of the left subclavian artery. Clamping of the proximal aorta will cause a rise in the BP, but not nearly as dramatic a rise as in patients with thoracic aneurysms because of the above mentioned collaterals. The more severe the "coarc" the less rise in BP with clamping because of more extensive collaterals. The BP can usually be controlled by deepening the anesthesia, although the addition of nitroprusside may be necessary. If there is concern about the blood supply to the spinal cord, moderate hypothermia - 32°C may be employed. The usefulness of this has not been established, but paraplegia is such a disastrous postop complication that we personally employ moderate hypothermia in this situation.

Before the surgeon releases the cross clamps, adequate volume replacement is absolutely necessary if profound hypotension is to be avoided.

Following completion of the operation, when the patient begins to awaken from anesthesia, severe hypertension may occur (7). Potent antihypertensive agents may be required. The etiology of the post-repair hypertension is not well understood at the present time.

Phrenic nerve injury may also occur intraoperatively with subsequent diaphragmatic paralysis (8).

The following conditions require extracorporeal circulation for repair, and some of the more common defects will be reviewed.

ASD

Children with uncomplicated atrial septal defects are classified as having non-cyanotic heart disease because of the tendency to shunt blood from left to right. There are two major types of ASD's.

The ostium secundum defect is simply a persistent foramen ovale and is located high in the septum. These patients are generally asymptomatic. The defects are usually closed to prevent pulmonary hypertension, to lessen the likelihood of SBE, or to prevent paradoxical emboli. Closure is either by a simple stitch or a pericardial or synthetic patch graft.

The ostium primum defect is much rarer and consists of a large defect in the inferior portion of the septum. In addition, a cleft mitral valve is a common associated finding. These patients routinely have increased pulmonary blood flow. Surgical repair is done to prevent irreversible pulmonary hypertension and cardiac failure.

Anesthesia for a patient with ostium secundum defect is straight forward. Remember, bubbles in all lines need to be meticulously avoided. Patients usually do well and there are few complications related to the repair.

A patient with an ostium primum defect offers a bigger challenge. If the systemic pressure decreases or the pulmonary pressure increases, the shunt may reverse with subsequent hypoxemia and profound bradycardia. Following repair, complete heart block is a well recognized complication. The P-R interval may lengthen, but usually produces no hemodynamic instability. The surgeon may perform a mitral valvuloplasty. When coming off bypass the surgeon may ask about the presence of a prominent "V" wave in order to evaluate any residual mitral incompetence.

VSD

Ventricular septal defect is the most common congenital heart defect found in children (6). Anatomic location in the septum is variable. The most common VSD lesion occurs in the membraneous septum just below the aortic valve. There can be a muscular defect in the lower portion of the septum. The muscular defects can also be multiple. Many small VSD's close spontaneously during the first year of life.

A patient with a VSD has left to right flow with the pulmonary blood flow increasing up to 4-5 times that of the systemic flow. The patient may go into pulmonary edema because of the increased flow. In infants, pulmonary artery banding may be done to decrease the flow (9). A pulmonary banding procedure may be technically difficult, and a band has been known to be placed on a branch of the pulmonary artery rather than on the main artery. If the band is placed too tightly, the patient may either slowly or abruptly deteriorate. This is heralded by bradycardia, hypotension, cyanosis, etc. Therefore, once the band is placed, the patient is observed for about ten minutes before proceeding. Once the patient is shown to tolerate the procedure, RV, PA, and LV pressures may be measured to check the effectiveness of the band. The PA pressure ideally should be about 1/2 or less than the systemic pressure. If the patient deteriorates after the band is placed, resuscitative measures are usually not successful until the band is removed.

At 2-5 years of age, the patient may return for his definitive VSD repair. The principles of anesthesia are primarily directed at avoiding a right to left shunt. The patient should be adequately premedicated, followed by low dose pentothal or ketamine, intubation, and light anesthesia for maintenance along with muscle relaxation, preferably pancuronium.

The correction is often performed through a right atrial approach, which produces less postop depression by not interfering with the integrity of the right ventricle. A membraneous defect closure may produce total heart block because of misplacement of a septal stitch. If the heart block is permanent, the patient will always require a pacemaker. The tricuspid or mitral valve may be compromised so that insufficiency results.

The routine patient following a VSD repair presents little problem in postop care, and early extubation is encouraged.

If the defects were multiple, a residual shunt may be present. In order to document this, a cardiogreen dye curve may be performed in the

ICU. If the defect produces hemodynamic instability, subsequent re-exploration may be necessary.

TETRALOGY OF FALLOT

Tetralogy of Fallot is a complex congenital heart syndrome consisting of a VSD, pulmonary stenosis, right ventricular hypertrophy, and overriding (dextroposition) of the aorta. The obstruction to flow from the right ventricle may occur at: infundibulum, pulmonic valve, annulus or pulmonary artery(ies).

Patients become progressively more cyanotic and may develop right heart failure. Frequently these children require a systemic to pulmonary artery shunt early in their lives to increase pulmonary blood flow. When they come for a total correction, one may see a severely cyanotic, small, polycythemic patient who has marked clubbing. These children give a history of frequently maintaining a squatting position because this maneuver increases peripheral vascular resistance and therefore increases the left to right shunt which increases the paO_2.

The induction of these patients requires an anesthetic technique which attempts to avoid right to left shunting. If such shunting should occur severe hypoxemia may produce marked bradycardia or even cardiac arrest. Heavy premedication is useful to prevent crying on induction. Bucking and straining are to be avoided. Ketamine is useful as an induction agent to increase systemic vascular resistance. Halothane may be used, but generally low doses are required to prevent a marked decrease in SVR, small doses of phenylephrine are pharmacologically indicated. Propranolol, 0.05 to 0.1 mg/k should be considered as an attempt to increase the size of the outflow tract. The rationale is similar to propranolol's use in patients with IHSS.

With marked polycythemia, hypothermia must be carefully assessed since a decrease in temperature will cause a marked rise in viscosity producing sludging and decreased perfusion to low flow organs. Hemodilution is very helpful.

Surgery is frequently difficult because the site of the pulmonary stenosis may not be the valve but rather the pulmonary artery/arteries. This area can be widened by using a patch graft often from the pericardium. This stenosis is often the limiting factor in the repair (10).

Complications of a total correction include:

1) Complete Heart Block
2) Residual Pulmonary Stenosis
3) Right Heart Failure

An important factor in the development of heart failure is the location of the cardiac incision. An incision in the right ventricle produces more myocardial dysfunction than one in the atrium. Postoperatively, monitoring the right atrial pressure may be more important than the left sided pressures, since right heart failure occurs more often than left.

TRANSPOSITION OF THE GREAT VESSELS (Mustard Operation)

A straight forward transposition has the aorta arising anteriorly from the right ventricle and the pulmonary trunk posteriorly from the left ventricle. Cyanosis is inversely related to the degree of shunt. Obviously, if no shunt exists, e.g. PDA, ASD, VSD, etc., the patient will die when the cord is clamped. If a shunt is present, cyanosis will intensify on crying, but not as much as in a tetralogy patient. It has been noted that children with transposition who have large ASD's will do quite well for a time. Palliative procedures have been developed based on this observation. A Rashkind (9) procedure is an atrial septostomy performed with a balloon catheter. In a Blalock-Hanlon operation, an ASD is surgically created.

Permanent correction is usually necessary by three years of age because of progressive cyanosis, polycythemia, and thromboembolic phenomena. The Mustard procedure involves excising the interatrial septum and constructing a baffle so that blood returning via the venae cavae goes to the left side and blood from the pulmonary veins is shunted to the right side. Thus, the right ventricle becomes the systemic ventricle. The operation may be unsuccessful if pulmonary hypertension is extremely advanced. The Rastelli operation (11) is used in patients with transposition of the great vessels and pulmonary stenosis. A Hancock conduit is placed between the right ventricle and the pulmonary artery.

Shunt reversal on induction needs to be avoided. Myocardial depression occurs readily because of the systemic right ventricle. Since polycythemia is severe, hypothermia needs to be induced along with hemodilution if thromboses are to be avoided. During the surgical repair total circulatory arrest (12) may be performed when the temperature reaches 10°C. Up to 60 minutes of total circulatory arrest seem to be tolerated quite well (13). The arrest is induced to provide a surgeon with a heart that is quiet and empty of blood. Both left and right atrial pressures are useful in postop management. Inotropic support is often necessary.

TRICUSPID ATRESIA (Fontan Operation)

A Fontan Operation (14) is performed for palliation of tricuspid atresia and consists of either a Hancock conduit or a tube graft from the right atrium to the pulmonary artery. In addition to the tricuspid atresia, the patients have a VSD, an ASD, or both and may have transposition of the great vessels. In infancy, the patients may have had a Blalock shunt because of inadequate pulmonary blood flow. These patients have a hypoplastic right ventricle and a huge right atrium.

When the patients arrive for the procedure, the Blalock shunt may be functioning. This is dissected free, but cannot be closed before bypass. Once bypass is initiated, the shunt has to be closed before ventricular fibrillation or asystole occurs or else blood will flood the lungs.

These patients are severely cyanotic with clubbing, polycythemia, etc. Since the operation connects one low pressure system (RT atrium) to another (PA), the patients are likely to have problems getting blood through the lungs postoperatively. Therefore, high LA pressures postop will lower the effective right sided driving pressure. In the face of low cardiac output, the LA pressure may actually have to be decreased rather than increased. Positive pressure ventilation as well as PEEP will predictably not be well tolerated. Extubation at the earliest indicated time should be planned.

These patients tend to bleed excessively. The graft needs to be pre-clotted and fresh frozen.

IHSS

Idiopathic hypertrophic subaortic stenosis may be seen in the neonatal, pediatric, young adult, or geriatric population. The clinical picture mimics aortic stenosis. Four mechanical problems are usual:

1) Outflow tract obstruction in one or both ventricles.
2) Impaired left ventricular filling or decreased left ventricular compliance secondary to LVH.
3) Mitral insufficiency is often present.
4) Decreased mechanical efficiency of the hypertrophied myocardium.

Basic mechanisms which can increase the obstruction are:
1) Increased contractility.
2) Decreased preload.
3) Decreased afterload.

Hypotension should not be treated with:
1) Digitalis
2) Ca^{++}
3) Beta I Agonists

The above increase contractility and worsen the outflow obstruction.

The classical pharmacologic treatment is:
1) Propranolol and/or
2) Verapamil (15)

Amyl Nitrate, Nitroglycerin, and Nitroprusside make matters worse. Squatting lessens the murmur. For anesthetic management remember:
a) Keep the heart full and dilated.
b) Avoid hypovolemia, veno and arterial vasodilation.

Surgical septectomy is the operation of choice done on total bypass. The induction and intraop periods are difficult because of recurrent hypotension; postop there are few problems unless surgical complications have occurred.

There are a myriad of congenital cardiac anomalies which are impossible to remember. Therefore, it is necessary to look up the anatomy prior to the planned surgical procedure. Many times the anatomy found at the time of surgery differs from the cath interpretation.

Always be prepared for the worst: during ligation of a PDA, should the patient become very hypertensive and develop pulmonary edema, perhaps the descending thoracic aorta was ligated by mistake. Intraoperatively, it is absolutely necessary to watch the surgical field so that surgical displacement of the heart, compression of the lungs, or kinking of the great vessels may be readily appreciated. Bradycardia is

64

a warning sign suggesting hypoxemia of the heart itself and is the precursor of cardiac arrest.

There is no more difficult psychological problem confronting an anesthesiologist than having one of these babies die, either intraoperatively or in the ICU. One needs to steel oneself to remain "unattached" to these children if depression is to be avoided.

Finally, there is very little written about anesthesia for congenital heart disease because the individual lesions are quite rare and large series are difficult to acquire. Thus, one's approach needs to be:

a) Understand the anatomy

b) understand the direction and amount of blood flow under various conditions

c) select anesthetic agents, techniques, vasopressors, etc. based upon "b"

d) calculate correctly drug dosages before the case begins

e) be vigilant

f) Primum, non nocere.

REFERENCES

1. Bini, M., Reves, J.G., et al. Anesth. Analg. 63:186, 1984.
2. Hickey, P.R., and Hansen, D.H. Anesth. Analg. 63:117-124, 1984.
3. Tarhan, Sait. Cardiovascular Anesthesia and Postoperative Care. Year Book Medical Publishers, Inc., Chicago, Ill. 1982.
4. Bhat, R., Fisher, E., et al. Pediatric Clinics of North America 29:1117, 1982.
5. Mikhail, M., Lee, W., Toeros, W., et al. J. Thorac. Cardiovasc. Surg. 83:349, 1982.
6. Braunwald, Eugene, Ed.: Heart Disease. W.B. Saunders, Co., Philadelphia, PA, 1980.
7. Fisher, A., Benedict, C.R. Anaesthesia 32:533, 1977.
8. Lynn, A.M., Jenkins, J.G., et al. Crit. Care Med. 11:280, 1983.
9. Stewart, S., et al. J. Thorac. Cardiovasc. Surg. 80:431, 1980.
10. Blackstone, E.H., Kirklin, J.W. and Pacifico, A.D. J. Thorac. Cardiovasc. Surg. 77:526, 1979.
11. Rastelli, G.C., McGoon, D.C. and Wallace, R.B. J. Thorac. Cardiovasc. Surg. 58:545, 1969.
12. Bailey, L.L., Takeuchi, Y., et al. J. Thorac. Cardiovasc. Surg. 71:485, 1976.
13. Wells, F.C., Coghill, S., et al. J. Thorac. Cardiovasc. Surg. 86:823, 1983.
14. Gale, A.W., Danielson, G.K., et al. J. Thorac. Cardiovasc. Surg. 78:831, 1979.
15. Rosing, D.R., Kent, K.M., et al. Circulation 60:1201, 1979.

ANESTHETIC CONSIDERATIONS FOR CEREBRAL VASCULAR SURGERY

J. D. MICHENFELDER

Surgery for occlusive cerebrovascular disease can be classified
into two major categories: extracranial (primarily carotid
endarterectomy), and extra- to intracranial anastomosis (for example,
superficial temporal artery to middle cerebral artery).

CAROTID ENDARTERECTOMY
For carotid endarterectomy, the major goals for proper anesthetic
management are twofold: 1) to use monitoring techniques that will
detect the onset of cerebral ischemia during carotid occlusion and 2)
to use anesthetic agents and techniques that will not aggravate but,
instead, prolong the tolerance of the brain for any ischemia that may
occur.
Monitoring
Possible approaches for monitoring these patients are summarized
in Table 1. Regional anesthesia (for example, deep cervical block)

Table 1
MONITORING CEREBRAL OXYGENATION
Avoid general anesthesia
Cerebral perfusion pressure
Cerebral blood flow
Cerebral metabolism
Cerebral function

would permit continuous monitoring of the patient's neurologic
function during the entire surgical procedure and, thus, would permit
the immediate detection of cerebral ischemia. However, this is the
preferred method of only a small number of surgeons and
anesthesiologists. Objections include patient discomfort, inability
to use "protective" techniques, and perhaps most importantly, the
potential for panic on the part of the patient, surgeon, and
anesthesiologist should a neurologic deficit occur during the
procedure. In this regard, it should be noted that onset of a
neurologic deficit due to incomplete focal ischemia in no way implies

an irreversible process; with return of an adequate cerebral circulation, return of normal function has been observed even when the ischemic deficit has persisted for several hours.

When general anesthesia is used (as is most common), some type of indirect monitoring is indicated. Measurement of CBF would seem a logical and most appropriate monitor. However, that technology is rather complex and the equipment is expensive, such that with the exception of a few centers these measurements are not currently made.

The most commonly monitored variable is the cerebral perfusion pressure as reflected by the stump pressure. Stump pressure is that pressure measured distal to the surgically occluded carotid artery. It is therefore presumed to equal the collateral perfusion pressure via the circle of Willis. As commonly used, the critical stump pressure is considered to be 50 mmHg, above which flow is considered adequate, below which a shunt is considered necessary. Since knowledge of pressure alone cannot accurately predict flow (without knowledge of resistance as well) this might be expected to be a relatively crude monitor of the adequacy of cerebral oxygenation. This relationship was studied in a series of patients undergoing carotid endarterectomy. The correlation between CBF and stump pressure was poor. However, in only 8% of the patients was stump pressure erroneous on the unsafe side; that is, the stump pressure was above the critical value of 50 mmHg and the CBF was below the critical value of 18 to 24 ml/100g/min. Perhaps a critical stump pressure of 60 mmHg would be a safer guideline for determining the need for a shunt if this is the only available monitor. One might well conclude from this study that, although stump pressure is far from perfect, it is better than no monitor at all.

Cerebral Metabolism. Another theoretical approach to monitoring the adequacy of cerebral oxygenation would be to measure some aspect of cerebral metabolism; for this purpose, jugular bulb blood oxygen levels were routinely monitored by many anesthesiologists up until the last decade. This fell out of favor when it was recognized that jugular bulb blood oxygen levels only reflect global cerebral oxygenation and could not be expected to detect regional ischemia as may be produced by occlusion of a single carotid artery.

Electroencephalogram. Finally, one might consider some aspect of cerebral function in the anesthetized patient. The only established approach is electroencephalography. Possibly in the future, monitoring an evoked response will become the preferred approach. Monitoring of a standard 16-lead electroencephalogram (EEG) is cumbersome and requires the continuous attention of a knowledgeable individual for interpretation. It is, therefore, expensive as well. In order to interpret the EEG, it must be artifact free and the

patient's anesthetic depth, carbon dioxide levels, and brain
temperature must be constant. Simplified versions of the standard EEG
are now available. Objections to these include their excessive cost
and loss of sensitivity.

Among available devices, the Cerebral Function Monitor (CFM) is
the simplest and least expensive; it is probably also the least
sensitive. In comparing the CFM to a standard electroencephalogram
(Table 2), it was found to detect ischemic changes readily in nine of

Table 2
COMPARISON OF STANDARD EEG AND CFM DURING
CAROTID OCCLUSION IN 55 PATIENTS

	EEG	CFM
No ischemic changes	44	46
Ischemic changes	11	9
False positives	--	0
False negatives	--	2

11 patients who showed changes in the standard EEG. In the two
failures, the magnitude of change in the standard EEG was minimal and
perhaps of no clinical significance. There were no false positives in
this study. Thus, as with stump pressure, the CFM is not perfect, but
it is certainly better than no monitor at all.

Anesthetic Techniques

Assuming general anesthesia is to be used, is there a preferred
technique? Table 3 lists proposed methods of protecting the brain

Table 3
PROPOSED TECHNIQUES FOR PROTECTING ISCHEMIC BRAIN
Insertion of shunt
Deep general anesthesia
Induced hypertension
Hypothermia
Hypercapnia
Hypocapnia
Hyperbaric oxygen

from ischemia. All but one of these proposed methods (insertion of a
shunt) are the primary responsibility of the anesthesiologist and
should therefore be examined in some detail.

General Anesthesia. Deep general anesthesia has long been
proposed and, most recently, specifically barbiturate-induced
anesthesia. There is consistent experimental evidence in animals that
barbiturates administered prior to establishing incomplete focal

cerebral ischemia will prolong the brain's tolerance for such ischemia. Accordingly, in the absence of adequate monitoring, it may well be appropriate to administer a "sleep dose" (3 to 5 mg/kg) of thiopental just prior to surgical occlusion of the carotid artery. This will produce near-maximal metabolic depression of the brain and, if there is severe ischemia following carotid occlusion, the thiopental effects should be prolonged because of lack of washout from these ischemic regions.

Cerebral protection might also be possible with isoflurane. At 2 MAC concentrations, it produces an isoelectric EEG and in animals a metabolic profile similar to that produced by barbiturates. Additional animal studies suggest protection with isoflurane from global incomplete ischemia but not from regional incomplete ischemia. In man we recently showed that the critical CBF (the CBF at which ischemic EEG changes occur) during light isoflurane anesthesia was as low as 8-10 ml/100g/min as compared to 18-24 ml/100g/min with light halothane or enflurane anesthesia. This implies a protective effect for isoflurane in man.

Because autoregulation is abolished by ischemia, many recommend the deliberate induction of mild hypertension during the period of carotid occlusion (20% above baseline). Thus, if there is ischemia during the period of carotid occlusion, any increase in pressure should result in some increase in flow to the ischemic area. This may be a hazardous technique in patients who also suffer from coronary artery disease, as is commonly the case in patients undergoing carotid endarterectomy. Monitoring a V_5 lead during the period of induced hypertension is recommended as a means of recognizing myocardial ischemia resulting from this intervention.

The use of either hypothermia or hyperbaric oxygen is primarily of historial interest; they have been essentially abandoned because of complexity, cost, and unexpected complications.

Hypercapnia versus Hypocapnia. Historically, both hypercapnia and hypocapnia have been recommended for patients undergoing carotid endarterectomy. Initially, hypercapnia was assumed to be effective until it was recognized that ischemic vessels do not respond to increasing carbon dioxide tensions (presumably they are already maximally dilated). It was then shown in animals that hypocapnia would, in fact, increase flow in ischemic areas by constricting the normal vasculature surrounding the ischemic region of brain. This, however, is a variable phenomenon and, in any given patient, the effect of a change in carbon dioxide in either direction on CBF is unknown. For this reason, it is now generally accepted that if a patient is neurologically stable at his normal $PaCO_2$ then that is the level at which the patient should be maintained during the course of the operative procedure.

From these considerations one can develop a reasonable recommendation for anesthetic management. Avoidance of hypotension during induction and maintenance of anesthesia is clearly critical (remember that autoregulation may be lost in these patients). Induction with thiopental is appropriate. Selection of agents for maintenance may be influenced by the planned monitoring. Thus, if the EEG is to be monitored, a constant anesthetic depth is most easily achieved using a volatile agent (plus nitrous oxide). Our current choice is isoflurane. There is no proven contraindication to the use of narcotics, although the resulting cerebral vasoconstriction might be considered undesirable (however, as with hypocapnia, this in theory might result in a reverse steal effect in the ischemic regions). Carbon dioxide levels should be monitored during the procedure and the patient should be maintained at normocapnia (this is, at his normal $PaCO_2$). The selective use of induced hypertension during carotid occlusion is recommended and, if a volatile agent is in use, this is probably best accomplished with an alpha agonist such as phenylephrine (to avoid ventricular irritability).

EXTRACRANIAL TO INTRACRANIAL VASCULAR ANASTOMOTIC PROCEDURES

The existing areas of cerebral ischemia for which these patients are undergoing surgery may be expected to have lost all capacity for autoregulation, and thus flow to these areas is totally pressure dependent. Maintenance of an adequate cerebral perfusion pressure at all times is perhaps the paramount consideration in these patients.

It is not uncommon during angiographic procedures in these patients to observe transient neurologic deficits that are titratable by alterations in blood pressure.

As with carotid endarterectomy patients, because of the unpredictable effects of changes in carbon dioxide on regional CBF in the presence of regional ischemia, it is important to maintain these patients during surgery at their normal carbon dioxide tension. Once again, there is no evidence to indicate a preference for either a volatile agent or a narcotic:nitrous oxide:relaxant technique. It should be noted that control of ICP is not a major concern in these patients, and therefore a volatile agent in combination with normocapnia is not contraindicated.

Again, an indication may exist for the use of thiopental in this procedure in the hope of protecting potentially ischemic brain. The procedure requires that the surgeon temporarily occlude a branch of the middle cerebral artery to which the superficial temporal artery is to be anastomosed. Thus, an unknown degree of ischemia may occur in the area of brain supplied by that small branch of the middle cerebral artery. Accordingly, before surgical occlusion of this branch, 3 to 5 mg/kg of thiopental may be desirable. Repeat doses are not given during the period of anastomosis since, if the area is ischemic, one could not deliver further thiopental to it. This is another example of thiopental therapy in a situation where it probably will do no harm and may well do some good.

Except for knowledge of blood gases and careful control of blood pressure, no unusual monitoring is required in these patients. Although these are generally high-risk patients, the surgical procedure itself is relatively minor, requiring only a small craniotomy and no brain dissection whatsoever. Thus, the risk is primarily anesthetic rather than surgical, and with adherence to proper anesthetic principles and attention to control of blood pressure and blood gases, the morbidity and mortality should be minimal. These procedures are surgically tedious in inexperienced hands and may require as long as 10 to 12 hours. With experience, this time should be decreased to less than four hours as a routine.

A recent prospective, randomized multi-institutional study of the efficacy of this surgical procedure failed to demonstrate any beneficial effects compared to unoperated controls. Accordingly, there is a concerted effort to force surgeons to abandon this procedure on the part of neurologists, the government, third party payers, and some neurosurgeons. Interestingly, the same individuals responsible for this study now hope to follow up with a randomized prospective study of the efficacy of carotid endarterectomy.

ANEURYSMS AND A-V MALFORMATIONS

In patients undergoing surgery for aneurysms or AV malformations the major concern is usually not cerebral ischemia but rather control of blood pressure so as to avoid inadvertent rupture of the aneurysm or excessive bleeding from the AV malformation. Adequate surgical exposure is also a critical requirement thus indicating the use of techniques that will reduce brain bulk. In addition to proper anesthetic selection this may include the use of such techniques as intravenous hyperosmotic agents and drainage of cerebral spinal fluid. For induction of hypotension we currently prefer either isoflurane alone or in combination with sodium nitroprusside. The concern regarding cyanide toxicity, although a real one, is easily avoided by limiting the total dose given the patient to 1 to 1.5 mg/kg. It is our clinical experience that the dose of nitroprusside required can be minimized by the use of anesthetics such as isoflurane. For these patients there is no absolute contraindications to the use of induced hypotension. The risk of not using hypotension generally overrides all other risk considerations. Based upon both experimental and human

work, it is reasonable to assume that a 30 percent reduction in the
patient's normal blood pressure will be tolerated without any
significant reduction in cerebral blood flow. If necessary, as much
as a 50 percent reduction in blood pressure may be used without a
major risk of cerebral ischemia although a significant reduction in
cerebral blood flow will occur at these pressure levels. Greater than
a 50 percent reduction in the patient's normal blood pressure may be
expected to result in a time related degree of cerebral ischemia. In
aneurysm surgery the major goal is to maintain a normal or reduced
transmural pressure across the wall of the aneurysm. Thus before the
surgeon opens the dura, a modest decrease in blood pressure should be
induced since the pressure outside of the aneurysm will be abruptly
decreased upon opening the dura. During manipulation of the aneurysm
a 30-40 percent reduction in arterial pressure is maintained and
should the aneurysm inadvertently rupture then profound degrees of
hypotension may be required for the surgeon to gain control. If one
anticipates the need for significant degrees of hypotension (greater
than 30-40% reduction) then it would be appropriate to consider a
prior dose of thiopental (3-5 mg/kg) with intermittent (every 5-10
min) small doses (1/2-1 mg/kg) during the period of hypotension.
Hypothermia which was once the preferred technique for aneurysm
surgery in many institutions has now largely been abandoned. The
techniques were largely complex and time consuming and introduced
complications of their own. With the introduction of the operating
microscope and the use of potent hypotensive agents, the morbidity and
mortality from aneurysm surgery has been greatly reduced.

REFERENCES

1. Sundt, T.M., Sharbrough, F.W., Anderson, R.E., et. al. J. Neurosurg. 41:310-320, 1974.
2. Boysen, G. Acta. Neurol. Scand. (Suppl 52) 49:1-84, 1973.
3. Easton, J.D. and Sherman, D.G. Stroke 8:565-568, 1977.
4. McKay, R.D., Sundt, T.M., Michenfelder, J.D., et. al. Anesthesiology 45:390-399, 1976.
5. Harp, J.R. and Wollman H. Br. J. Anaesth. 45:256-262, 1973.
6. Lassen, N.A. Circ. Res. 34:749-760, 1974.
7. Sharbrough, F.W., Messick, J.M. and Sundt, T.M. Stroke 4:674-684, 1973.
8. Moore, D.S. and Hall, A.D. Arch. Surg. 99:702-710, 1969.
9. Fourcade, H.E., Larson, C.P., Ehrenfeldt, W.K., et. al. Anesthesiology 33:383-390, 1970.
10. Sublett, J.W., Seidenberg, A.B. and Hobson, R.W. Anesthesiology 41:505-508, 1974.
11. Boysen, G., Ladegaard-Pedersen, H.J., Henriksen, H., et. al. Anesthesiology 35:286-300, 1971.
12. Casement, B., Messick, J.M., Milde, L., et. al. Anesthesiology 63:A406, 1985.
13. Michenfelder, J.D. The assessment of cerebral function. Can. Anaesth. Soc. J. 31:S13-S15, 1984.
14. Michenfelder, J.D. Clin. Neurosurg. 32:105-113, 1985.

CARE OF THE PACEMAKER PATIENT UNDERGOING GENERAL SURGERY

J. ZAIDAN

Increasingly complex permanent pacemakers are used in greater
numbers each year. The anesthesiologist, therefore, may care for these
patients who are scheduled for general surgery. This lecture will
acquaint the anesthesiologist with types of pacemakers, patient and
pacemaker evaluations, intraoperative management and pacemaker failure,
and indications for perioperative pacemaker insertion.

Types of pacemaker generators fall into two categories. The
asynchronous generator contains one circuit that creates and emits
impulses. This generator wastes energy and competes with the patient's
intrinsic conduction system. The synchronous pacemaker contains two
circuits: one that creates and emits impulses and a second circuit that
senses intrinsic depolarization. Synchronization eliminates competition
and in the ventricular inhibited pacemaker, conserves energy.

Evaluation of the patient is an important part of preoperative
care. These patients commonly have coronary artery disease,
hypertension, and diabetes mellitus and receive a variety of drugs that
should continue to surgery.(1, 2) These drugs include beta-blocking and
calcium channel blocking drugs, cardiac glycosides, antiarrhythmics, and
diuretics. Manage insulin as you would with any other diabetic.
Consider consulting a cardiologist when the patient has a return of
symptoms that led to pacemaker implantation. Determine if exercising
the muscles adjacent to the generator creates dizziness. This symptom
indicates that myopotentials inhibit the pacemaker.(3) This finding
implies that muscle fasciculations caused by succinylcholine and
shivering must be avoided.

Perform a general physical exam especially noting signs of
decreased ventricular performance, the presence of bruits, and the
location of the generator and leads.

The laboratory examination should minimally include an ECG, a chest x-ray, hemoglobin, and serum electrolytes. The guidelines for hemoglobin and electrolytes should be those which you normally accept for other surgical patients.

Pacemaker evaluation assumes secondary importance. Several very simple steps assure continued activity throughout surgery. If the patient's heart rate is slower than the pacing rate, then pacing spikes should appear on the ECG. To determine if these pacing impulses are associated with myocardial contractions, palpate a peripheral pulse. If each pacing impulse is not associated with a pulse, then consider a cardiology consult.

Evaluation of the pacemaker becomes more difficult when the patient's heart rate is greater than the pacing rate. A valsalva maneuver will slow the patient's rate so that pacing impulses will appear on the ECG. Carotid massage can potentially embolize an atherosclerotic plaque to the cerebral circulation, therefore avoid this technique. Generally, because sensing is lost before pacing, a pacing generator is probably functioning normally if it is less than two years old, if by chest x-ray the leads are intact, and impulses do not appear on the ECG.

Intraoperative management of the pacemaker patient can be complex, not because of the pacemaker, but because of the underlying disease. In general, the monitoring must be appropriate for the medical status of the patient. If, in your judgement, an IV, a blood pressure cuff, and an ECG are medically reasonable then do not insert an arterial catheter or a pulmonary arterial catheter. If, on the other hand, you believe that a pulmonary arterial catheter is necessary, then do not avoid its use. Document your reasons in the chart, especially if the patient has a transvenous electrode. All anesthetics have been successfully used in pacemaker patients. Anesthetic techniques include local, regional, and general. Use caution when selecting regional techniques in an anticoagulated patient. General techniques include inhalational and narcotic/relaxant. There exists no evidence that any of these anesthetic managements will alter pacemaker thresholds or sensing capabilities.

An important aspect of care of the pacemaker patient involves intraoperative failure of the pacemaker. Failure can be related to potassium equilibrium, electromagnetic interference, myopotentials, and myocardial ischemia and infarction.

The normal intracellular to extracellular potassium ratio is 30 to 1. This ratio results in a resting membrane potential of -90 millivolts. Acutely lowering this ratio by rapid potassium administration, myocardial ischemia leaking potassium to the extracellular space, or hypoventilation create a less negative resting membrane potential. The pacemaker with its constant output can more easily stimulate the myocardium to contraction and even cause ventricular tachycardia and fibrillation. The opposite occurs when the potassium ratio acutely rises. The resting membrane potential becomes more negative. Acute potassium loss and hyperventilation therefore cause loss of pacing capture.

The electrocautery is another cause of pacemaker failure. An asynchronous nonprogrammable generator (VOO or AOO) should not be inhibited by the electrocautery. The external generators can be adjusted to the asynchronous mode when the electrocautery is being used. Ventricular inhibited pacemakers (VIIO) revert to the asynchronous activity after they have turned off for one impulse. Programmable pacemakers can reprogram during electrocautery use if the magnet is placed over the generator. These generators can reprogram to virtually every possible mode of activity. If the generator has been programmed to asynchronous activity, it can simply reprogram out of asynchronous and become inhibited. For this reason, it is strongly recommended that the programmer be available if the generator converts to an activity that endangers the patient. All programmers contain a "panic button" that reprograms the generator to an output of 5 volts and a rate of 70 beats per minute in the ventricular inhibited mode.

Myopotentials inhibit pacemaker generators. The incidence varies from 10.8% to 85% in studies of nonanesthetized patients. (4, 5) Since signal amplitudes and slew rates of myopotentials overlap with those of intracardiac signals, the chance of pacemaker inhibition during muscle fasciculations caused by succinycholine administration or postoperative shivering is more than a theoretical possibility. One can circumvent this problem by reprogramming the generator to asynchronous (VOO) or by reprogramming to a less sensitive R-wave sensitivity. The generator still can be reprogrammed during the use of the electrocautery to something which would allow for inhibition by shivering in the postoperative period.

Myocardial infarction potentially can cause loss of pacing. (6) The current at the tip of the metal electrode provides a specific current density at the electrode-tissue interface. Scar tissue at this interface can conduct the current but it cannot be stimulated. The current will flow to the interface between the scarred tissue and tissue which can be stimulated. The presence of infarcted tissue around the metal electrode, therefore, effectively enlarges the electrode. If the same amount of current enters the metal electrode, the current density decreases at the infarcted tissue-stimulatable tissue interface. The stimulatable tissue, therefore, may not reach threshold causing loss of capture. The only method of reestablishing capture is to increase the output from the generator.

Clinical evidence indicates that the presence of an inhalational anesthetic does not acutely alter pacing thresholds. (7)

Indications for inserting a preoperative temporary electrode are judgemental. Suggested indications include extreme sinus bradycardia (atrial pacing), second or third degree A-V block (ventricular pacing), complete left bundle branch block before pulmonary artery catheterization (ventricular pacing), poorly controlled supraventricular dysrhythmias (atrial pacing), and bifascicular block combined with first degree A-V block when the patient has severe coronary artery disease (ventricular pacing). Consider the possibility of transcutaneous pacing rather than the invasive transvenous electrode.

Intra-atrial and intra-ventricular electrodes can be used to diagnose and then treat certain complex dysrhythmias. For instance, by recording the electrical impulses from within the atrium and comparing the atrial electrogram with a simultaneously recorded surface electrocardiogram, one can easily distinguish between atrial fibrillation and atrial flutter with varying block. Atrial flutter, along with other reentrant dysrhythmia can be terminated by rapid atrial pacing.(8) The ventricular electrode can be used to treat ventricular tachycardia.(9)

With careful preoperative preparation and watchful intraoperative care, the pacemaker patient should experience uneventful anesthesia and surgery. Remember that the pacemaker is not the problem. The real

problem is the underlying disease that necessitated pacemaker
implantation.

REFERENCES

1. Furman, S. Am Heart J 93:378, 1977.
2. Furman, S. Am Heart J 94, 1978.
3. Levine, P.A., Klein, M.D. Ann Int Med 98:101, 1983.
4. Piller, L.W., Lennelly, B.M. CHEST 66:418, 1977.
5. Ohm, O.J., Bruland, H., Pedersen, O.M., Waerness, E. Br Heart J
    36:77, 1974.
6. Tarjan, P. In: Cardiac Pacing (Eds. Samet, P., El-Sheif, N.). New
    York, 1980, pp. 89-110.
7. Zaidan, J.R., Curling, P.E., Craver, J.M. PACE 8:32, 1985.
8. Lister, J.W., Gosselin, A.J., Nathan, D.A., Barold, S.S. CHEST 63:
    995, 1973.
9. Fisher, J.D., Mehra, R., Furman, S. Am J Cardiol 41:94, 1978.

SUGGESTED READING

1. Zaidan, J.R. Anesthesiology 60:319, 1984.

ANESTHETIC CONSIDERATIONS IN PATIENTS FOR VASCULAR SURGERY

J. ARENS

Patients scheduled for vascular surgery procedures rarely have single organ or extremity involvement. The patients frequently are older men, moderately obese, moderately hypertensive, frequently diabetics who have involvement of multiple branches of aortic vessels including the carotid and coronary vessels. In addition, they are frequently on a multitude of drugs including antihypertensives, anticoagulants, hypoglycemics, antiarrhythmics, diuretics, etc.

Assessing risk is important if anesthetics and surgical procedures are to be varied and/or studied so that outcome of these patients undergoing various procedures can be improved.

Most studies involving risk are retrospective and therefore do not necessarily predict risk accurately for the preoperative group of patients. However, trends at least can be noted.

Goldman presented six primary preoperative factors which led to a high incidence of postoperative life threatening or fatal cardiac complications (1). These were:

A) S-3 Gallop or JVD.
B) Myocardial Infarction in preceeding 6 months.
C) Rhythm other than sinus, or PAC's on preop EKG.
D) >5 PVCs/min anytime preop.
E) Intraperitoneal, intrathoracic or aortic operation.
F) Age > 70 years.

Table 1. Risk Factors in 99 Patients Having Elective Aortic Surgery

	Number of Patients
History of smoking	97
Hypertension	55
Coronary artery disease	44
Previous myocardial infection (by history or ECG)	32
Angina	27
Previous CHF	10
Chronic respiratory disease	46
Diabetes	9
Renal impairment	3

Table 2. Serious Postoperative Cardiac Complications

	Number of Patients
Pulmonary edema	5
Myocardial infarction	5
Ventricular tachycardia	1
Cardiac death	1*

* Resulted from myocardial infarction.

Table 3. Comparison of Cardiac Complications in Two Groups

	Abdominal Aortic Patients		Goldman et al. Group		
Class	Number of Patients	Cardiac Complications	Number of Patients	Cardiac Complications	p*
1	56	4 (7%)	537	5 (1%)	0.01
2	35	4 (11%)	316	21 (7%)	NS
3	8	3 (38%)	130	18 (14%)	NS
TOTAL	99	11 (12%)	983	44 (4%)	0.01

* Pearson's chi-square and likelihood ratio chi-square of abdominal aortic patients vs. Goldman's group.

It is also known that coronary disease places a patient at higher risk. Patients with a previous M.I. have a greater likelihood of having another M.I. with surgery; the mortality from the 2nd M.I. is very high; M.I.'s most often occur on the 3rd postop day for reasons clearly not well understood.

When surgery is performed within 3 months of an M.I., the chance of reinfarction is 37%; at 3-6 months 16%; and from then on about 5%. The postop infarction patients have a mortality rate of 50-69% (3).

Crawford (4) has shown merely that patients who have had an infarction followed by CABG surgery have the same risk as those patients who have no coronary disease. Therefore, except in unusual circumstances, if a patient requires a vascular surgery procedure and a CABG operation, the CABG should be done first.

Tarhan has also shown that the incidence of postop myocardial infarction is related to the site of surgery (increased risk in upper abdominal and thoracic procedures).

What does one look for in the preoperative assessment? First of all, one needs to assess the cardiovascular reserve. A good history, therefore is paramount. However, assessing exercise tolerance in patients with claudication is obviously a problem.

A) Cutler has nicely pointed out the value of exercise testing in patients with peripheral vascular disease. Thirty-two vascular procedures were performed in patients with no EKG evidence of ischemia during testing, and no one infarcted or died. Sixteen patients showed exercise ischemia and 6 had postop M.I.'s, two of which were fatal. He urges such testing to:

1) assess severity of CAD and the likelihood of postop complications and,
2) use as a precautionary measure to identify potentially dangerous dysrhythmias in ischemia during exercise before clinical symptoms develop.

In addition, one learns:

1) The maximum pulse rate before ischemia occurs,
2) the pressure rate product at which ischemia occurs and,
3) which EKG lead best identifies the ischemic area.

B) In the latest CASS report (6), it has been shown that congestive heart failure is one of two variables which affect operative mortality. The other is emergency operation. Therefore, the presence or absence of CHF is determined by:

1) History
2) Physical - increased pulse, wheezing, pulsus alternans, JVD, gallops, etc.
3) EKG and X-ray evidence of a big heart.
4) Cath data if available.

If CHF is documented, then digitalization seems indicated. This is preoperative digitalization for CHF, and I do not consider this prophylactic. The question of prophylactic digitalization is still being debated.

C) Some assessment of respiratory function is necessary - these patients smoke, are obese, etc. If you aren't going to change your care because of pulmonary function tests, don't use them; if you do, utilize the "box" as well as ABG's. Preop teaching of the patient to breathe and cough effectively postop is very useful.

Management of a patient for abdominal aortic aneurysm surgery will now be discussed. If a patient has an aneurysm he should have surgery because of the possibility of rupture and/or dissection.

What monitors should be used?

A) EKG - preferably Lead V5 - to diagnose ischemia as well as arrhythmia.

B) A-Line - for obvious reasons - may be difficult to place because of severe peripheral vascular disease.

C) CVP at least, if no ischemia or CHF.

D) Swan-Ganz catheter if the patient has significant myocardial ischemia or congestive heart failure (poor left ventricular function). All patients for an abdominal aneurysmectomy do not need a Swan-Ganz. All patients for an abdominal aneurysmectomy should not be done with no patient getting a Swan-Ganz (7).

How is a Swan-Ganz especially helpful?

1) Induction - especially intubation.

2) Aortic X-clamping.

3) Early signs of volume depletion.

4) Aortic declamping.

5) Postop volume replacement.

6) Accurately determine coronary perfusion pressure.

One of the first group of patients that Drs. Gabel and Cevetta studied to show the value of a Swan-Ganz catheter in detecting disparate ventricular function were patients underlying abdominal aneurysmectomy. Cullen has shown a significant elevation of wedge pressure on aorta cross clamping and has in large part been responsible for popularizing the use of nitroprusside to decrease the afterload (8).

Aortic declamping has been a popular subject for many years. Simplistically, essentially all of the deleterious effects of declamping can be attributed to hypovolemia by suddenly increasing the size of the vascular bed and by the previously ischemic vascular bed becoming more permeable to fluids upon reperfusion, as well as the bed having diminished vascular tone. To avoid the hypotension, one should try to be the equivalent of one to two units of blood ahead (or an equivalent of a liter of white blood) and to encourage the surgeon to release the x-clamp slowly and to reclamp if necessary.

Popular explanations for hypotension have been:

A) Sudden release of metabolites - acidosis.

B) Hyperkalemia.

C) Release of myocardial depressant factors, etc. While all these may be possible, their clinical relevance is miniscule.

Abdominal aneurysms need to be done electively. The mortality rate for surgical correction of leaking aneurysm is quoted minimally at 25%. Back Pain in a preop abdominal aneurysm patient means dissection; in a postop patient means bleeding!!!

The postop complications which occur in aneurysm patients may affect one's anesthetic management (9):

A) Postop bleeding - already mentioned.

B) Colon ischemia - more common in emergency aneurysm surgery - due to direct injury - severe hypotension intraop, however, is probably not curative!

C) Renal dysfunction - obviously is more of a problem if the clamp has to go above the renal arteries.

D) Hypertension (10)

It needs to be stressed that intuitively one believes that repeated subclinical insults may have a significant additive effect on function renal reserve. Patients for this surgery may have diminished preoperative functional reserve because of age, intrinsic renal disease, arteriolar compromise due to hypertension or diabetes mellitus, or impaired perfusion due to CHF or renal artery atherosclerosis. This diminished functional reserve will increase the risk of clinical renal insufficiency if additional insults are sustained during the perioperative period (11).

Table 4. Clinical Setting for Renal Injury

Preoperative setting
  Nephrotoxic agents
    Iodinated contrast media
    Antibiotics
  Renal ischemia
    Volume contraction of extracellular fluid due to fasting, osmotic
      diuretics, bowel preparation, long-term diuretic therapy
Intraoperative setting
  Nephrotoxic agents
    Anesthetic agents, antibiotics
    Globin pigments (transfusion reaction, muscle necrosis)
  Renal ischemia
    Anesthetic agents
    Renal artery anatomic abnormalities (require clamping)
    Renal artery emboli
    Anti-prostaglandin synthetase medications
    Hemodynamic stress (hemorrhage, aortic clamping and unclamping,
      inappropriate volume replacement)
    Extracellular fluid sequestration (trauma, tissue ischemia)
Postoperative setting
  Nephrotoxic agents
  Renal ischemia
  Ureteral obstruction due to surgery

Renal failure during aortic surgery is primarily caused by renal ischemia. Renal autoregulation occurs between MAP of 80 to 160 mmHg. I can find little to document reflex vasoconstriction above the x-clamp as a cause of decreased renal perfusion. The surgical literature also supports the concepts of volume expansion and maintenance of hemodynamic stability. The use of 5% mannitol during cross clamping is primarily intuitive. The use of loop diuretics is the same except for the fact that these diuretics increase renal blood flow by stimulating the release of intrarenal prostaglandin-E (PGE) a potent dilator of afferent renal arterioles. Interestingly, this effect is blocked by preoperative administration of nonsteroidal anti-inflammatory agents, e.g. Indocin. In a series by McCombs (12), acute renal failure occurred in 2½% of patients following an elective resection whereas 21% of those undergoing an emergency repair developed acute renal failure.

The mortality rate in those patients who develop high output renal failure is 0% while the rate of those with oliguric renal failure is 70%.

E) Spinal cord ischemia - occurs in abdominal aneurysm surgery in about 0.25% of patients. Can't predict when this will occur.

F) Myocardial ischemia - in one group of patients, 57% with

abdominal aneurysm had clinically evident coronary artery disease, while 35% of patients with aorto-iliac disease had CAD. Those are sobering figures (13).

Table 5. Principal Causes of Operative Death After Aortic Reconstruction in 557 Patients at the Cleveland Clinic, 1974-1978 (data from Diehl et al.)

Principal cause of death	Intact AAA (n = 350)		Ruptured AAA (n = 34)		ASO (n = 173)	
	n	%	n	%	n	%
Myocardial infarction	11	3.1	3	8.8	3	1.7
Retroperitoneal bleeding	2	0.6	3	8.8	0	-
Sepsis	2	0.6	0	-	0	-
Multisystem failure	1	0.3	1	2.9	0	-
Renal failure	1	0.3	0	-	0	-
Congestive heart failure	0	-	1	2.9	0	-
Pulmonary failure	1	0.3	0	-	0	-
Pulmonary embolism	0	-	1	2.9	0	-
Stroke	0	-	0	-	1	0.6
Total	18	5.1	9	26.5	4	2.3

Table 6. Preoperative Cardiac Status, Postoperative Myocardial Infarction, and Mortality for 557 Patients Who Had Aortic Reconstruction at the Cleveland Clinic, 1974-1978 (data from Diehl et al.)

Preoperative cardiac status		Postoperative Myocardial Infarction		Operative Death	
	n	n	%	n	%
Negative cardiac history and normal ECG	210	2	1.4	6	2.9
CAD suspected either by history or ECG	193	12	6.2	10	5.2
CAD suspected both by history and ECG	154	14	9.1	15	9.7
Total	557	29	5.2	31	5.6

G) Lower limb anesthesia - primarily a surgical complication.

ANESTHETIC MANAGEMENT

An anesthetic technique for this operation should embody the following principles:

A) Amnesia and adequate analgesia

B) Abolish noxious reflexes

C) Decrease MVO_2

D) Minimal cardiovascular depression

E) Relatively short acting

The anesthetic one would use for anesthetizing a "sick heart" is appropriate. A word of caution needs to be made regarding the use of muscle relaxants. Remember, the cardiovascular effects of the relaxant and choose accordingly. However, also remember the mode of elimination. If the aneurysm extends above the renals, a relaxant which is primarily eliminated through the kidneys is perhaps not a good choice.

In a yet unpublished study, El Etr (14) of Chicago showed that patients with recent M.I.'s who were anesthetized by cardiac anesthetists as if they were having CABG surgery did not have a higher infarction rate than the normal population. This is certainly encouraging.

The use of spinal or epidural anesthesia is controversial because:

A) Duration of procedure

B) Extent of procedure

C) Anti-coagulation (15)

D) Associated coronary and cerebral artery disease

E) Sudden volume shifts

Recovery room problems may be multiple with these patients.

A) Ventilation is critical. These patients are often best left intubated until they meet documented extubation criteria.

B) Blood Pressure Control is a major problem.

1) Hypertension is frequently a major problem, and preop antihypertensives need to be reinstituted as soon as possible. Nipride is effective for the short term, but other agents should be employed if Nipride is used in large quantities or for a long period of time.

2) Hypotension may be due to bleeding, sequestration of fluid into retroperitoneal space, over-enthusiastic usage of diuretics, etc. Obviously, myocardial causes need also be considered.

C) Hypothermia needs to be corrected slowly, since tissue perfusion is often poor and burns are readily produced by warming blankets, etc.

D) Circulation to legs needs to be assessed frequently in the recovery room.

E) Renal function needs to be monitored carefully.

The management of other lower limb peripheral vascular surgical procedures is quite similar although not quite so complex because of the absence of cross clamp and declamp problems. However, the surgery is technically difficult and often very tedious. Often the vascular disease is more diffuse and extensive. The peripheral nature of the surgery often makes us take down our guard.

Anesthesia for a thoracic aneurysm is as involved as anything else in our specialty. The patients are often quite elderly and often poorly worked-up because of the sudden onset of symptoms. Often the patient has uncontrolled hypertension, since this hypertension has caused the aneurysm to expand. When evaluating the patient for surgery, it is helpful to determine the location as well as size of the aneurysm. Specific points need to be made about the management.

A) Two A-lines are necessary:
   1) in the right radial - the aneurysm may involve the left subclavian.
   2) a femoral line - discuss which side with the surgeon - use side opposite from where perfusion of lower body will be performed.
B) Use of double lumen tube - use left sided tube - left lung is manipulated by surgeon during repair and before use of double lumen tubes, postop the left lung was "whited out" because of intra-parenchymal hemorrhage.
C) Need to be prepared to manage severe hypertension when the surgeon x-clamps proximal aorta. Inhalational agents are helpful and vasodilators will likely be needed.
D) Kidney protection needs to be emphasized. Adequate perfusion is of paramount importance, but other techniques such as isotonic mannitol, furosemide, dopamine may afford some good.
E) Extent of proximal dissection - e.g. cerebral blood supply - aortic valve involvement does have implications. The same is true of distal dissection - involvement of celiac artery, renal arteries, etc.

A thoracic aneurysm may present as a mass, with "tearing" chest pain due to dissection, as a stroke, as aortic insufficiency or as a left sided hemothorax.

During the resection of the thoracic aneurysm, the surgeon will clamp the aorta just above and below the aneurysm. If the aneurysm is in the classical location - distal to the left subclavian artery - the heart itself will provide perfusion to the head and the rest of the upper body. However, the lower half of the body will be without a blood supply. There are four basic techniques to perfuse the distal portion:

A) A graft may be run from the subclavian artery to the femoral artery. The advantage is that total heparinization need not be used and there is no need for the pump. However, the flow rate of blood in this graft is often low and the distal pressure poor. A Gott Shunt is used.

B) Extracorporeal Circulation can be used - blood is pumped into the femoral artery and removed via the femoral vein. Total heparinization is required, but flow rates are easily controlled. However, if the "systemic pulsatile pressure" begins to decrease, to increase the BP the pump must be <u>slowed</u> rather than increased because increasing flow actually siphons more blood into the reservoir and may produce a hypovolemic pressure and even cardiac arrest.

C) Left Heart Bypass - left atrial to femoral artery - may be performed with one pump head, and regional heparinization may be employed. However, in this area of the country, this technique is uncommon.

D) In many institutions, the thoracic aorta is merely clamped and surgery is performed rapidly to decrease the time of distal ischemia. Additionally, in some institutions, the adjunct of moderate hypothermia may be also employed.

Because of the extent and duration of the surgery, the incidence of postoperative complications is very high. Some of the more commonly seen complications include:

A) Stroke

B) Intraop Hypertension secondary to clamping aorta. Following clamping of the proximal aorta, severe hypertension can occur. The BP needs to be treated to prevent:

1) stroke

2) heart failure

3) clamp slipping off aorta.

Because of the precarious status of many of these patients,

nitroprusside is probably a better choice than propranolol, though obviously it is difficult for the Nipride to dilate a steel clamp on the aorta.

C) Post-op bleeding - especially suture line.

D) Hypoxemia secondary to hemorrhage into the up lung. The hypoxemia results from the surgeon handling the "up" lung with hemorrhage to that lung as a consequence. Thus, it is recommended that a double lumen tube be placed so that complete collapse of the lung can be produced.

E) Paraplegia - the radicularis magna artery comes off at T7 and in some patients provides the majority of blood supply to the cord (16, 17). The incidence of paraplegia is about 7% in all series including series for traumatic as well as atherosclerotic lesions. There have been no prospective studies done, so the problem has not really been resolved. If the blood supply to the cord in a particular patient is truly segmental rather than confluent, little probably can be done to prevent paraplegia. Remember, elevation of venous pressure as well as ICP will decrease spinal cord perfusion pressure and need to be avoided if possible.

F) Renal dysfunction secondary to impaired renal perfusion.

G) Intestinal ischemia or necrosis. Postop, a persistent early rise in K^+ should alert one to such a possibility.

H) Hypothermia - if shivering is either prevented or attenuated in the postop period, some of the serious consequences of hypothermia will be avoided. However, with hypothermia, the following may occur:

1) CNS depression secondary to the cold.

2) Increased solubility of the inhalational agents.

3) Diminished ventilation requirements due to decreased CO_2 production.

4) Shift of CO_2 response curve to the right.

5) Potentiation of muscle relaxants.

6) Increased blood viscosity especially with an elevated Hct.

7) Shift of oxyhemoglobin curve to the left.

When discussing vascular surgery procedures, the subject of amputation arises. After a series of vascular operations in patients with severe peripheral as well as systemic vascular disease, the operations may all fail and an amputation of a portion of the lower limb will be necessary. By this time, the patient may have become more sick than when he was originally scheduled for the major vascular surgery procedure.

Risk - The risk in this group of patients is awful. As you can see in the Figure produced from Poulsen et al. (18) there is a linear relationship to the site of surgery as well as to age. I'm not sure how or if we need to change management of these cases, but the mortality figures are startling, to say the least.

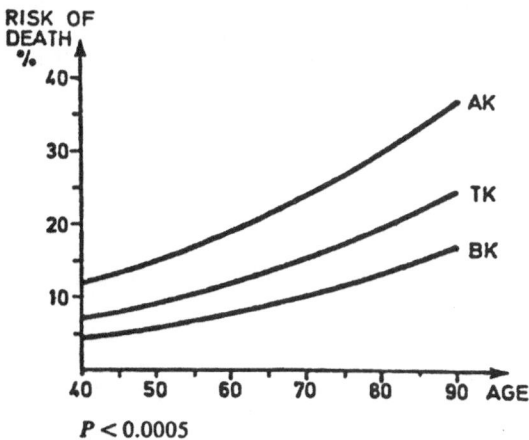

$P < 0.0005$

Figure 3. Estimated probability of death during hospitalization in relation to age.

The choices of anesthesia can include:
A) General
B) Intravenous agents alone or in combination
C) Spinal or epidural
D) Sciatic-femoral block
E) Regional hypothermia

If one were to do an AK amputation with peripheral nerve blocks, four nerves require blocking - e.g. sciatic, femoral, obturator, and lateral femoral cutaneous nerves. This would require a large quantity of local anesthetics which would be near or in excess of the toxic dose.

REFERENCES

1. Goldman, L., et al. Medicine 57:357, 1978.
2. Jeffrey, C.C., Cullen, D.J., et al. Anesthesiology 58:462, 1983.
3. Stein, P.A., Tinker, J.H., and Tarhan, S. JAMA 239:2566, 1978.
4. Crawford, E.S., et al. Ann. Thorac. Surg. 26:215, 1978.
5. Cutler, B.S., et al. Am. J. Surg. 137:484, 1979.
6. Miller, D.C., et a. J. Thorac. Cardiovasc. Surg. 85:197, 1983.
7. Attia, R.R., et a. (Mass General). Circulation 53:961, 1976.
8. Cullen, D.J., Silverstein, P., et al. Anesthesiology 50:462, 1979.
9. Crawford, E.S. Surgery 93:91, 1983.
10. Grindlinger, G.A., et al. Am. J. Surg. 141:472, 1981.
11. Bush, H.L. Surg. 93:107, 1983.
12. McCombs. S.G.O. 148:176, 1979.
13. Hertzer, Norman. Surgery 93:97, 1983.
14. Rao, T.L.K., EL-Etr, R. Anesth. Analg. 60:271-272, 1981 (Abstract).
15. Odoom, J.A. Anaesthesia 38:254, 1983.
16. Costello, T.G., and Fisher, A. Anaesthesia 38:230, 1983.
17. Conti, V.R., Calverly, J., et al. Ann. Thorac. Surg. 33:81, 1982.
18. Mandrup-Poulsen, T., and Jensen, J.S. Acta Orthop. Scand. 53:879, 1982.

PROTECTING THE BRAIN DURING AND AFTER VASCULAR INSUFFICIENCY

J. D. MICHENFELDER

After years of controversy and hosts of animal studies, the issue
of barbiturate brain protection has been largely resolved based upon
valid human studies which are supported by animal studies. Despite an
initial enthusiastic endorsement by many clinicians, it can now be
stated unequivocally that there is no place for barbiturate therapy
following resuscitation from cardiac arrest. This was established in
a prospective, randomized, multi-institutional trial in man which
failed to demonstrate even a suggestion that barbiturates might
favorably alter neurologic outcome.(1) Further this same result has
been reported in all of the recent animal studies that addressed this
question.(2-4) One presumed explanation for these negative results is
simply that cerebral metabolic suppression by barbiturates (and other
anesthetics) is not possible in the absence of an active EEG. The
latter can be expected to remain isoelectric for many minutes
following resuscitation.

By contrast in the event of incomplete ischemia, EEG activity is
usually present (albeit altered) and metabolic suppression and hence
possibly protection can be induced with barbiturates. Indeed, most of
the animal studies which have addressed this question have been
positive in that barbiturates improve the brain's tolerance for the
ischemic insult as judged by whatever index was being used (metabolic,
electrophysiologic, histopathologic, or outcome).(5-7) These
consistent results led to a number of recommendations for barbiturate
therapy in man for incomplete ischemia. These included during carotid
occlusion for carotid endarterectomy, during temporary occlusion of
intracranial cerebral arteries for aneurysm and by-pass procedures,
during profound hypotension and during cardiopulmonary bypass. The
last of these suggested indications was subjected to a prospective
randomized trial in man by Nussmeier et al.(8) Their results were
unambiguous: patients given large doses of thiopental during bypass
(approximately 3 g) had no neuro-psychiatric deficits on the tenth
postoperative day while in the control patients there was a
significant incidence of 7.5%. All of the patients in this study were
undergoing procedures that required an open ventricle since this is

associated with a greater incidence of neuropsychiatric disorders (presumably embolic). The authors recommendation to adopt such therapy seems appropriate. However, it has been postulated that since they used normothermic perfusion, bubble oxygenators, and no arterial filters that the control group had an exaggerated incidence of deficits which magnified the beneficial effects of thiopental. This does not challenge the scientific validity of the study but rather the appropriateness of such therapy if hypothermia, membrane oxygenators and filters are used. It should be noted, however, that their reported incidence of deficits of 7.5% in the control group does not appear to be excessive when compared to the incidence reported for other groups of patients undergoing cardiopulmonary bypass.(9-11) In any case their valid demonstration of bariburate induced brain protection in man gives credibility to the other suggested indications for barbiturate therapy as summarized above.

A third possible indication for barbiturate therapy is in head trauma. Here again a recent randomized prospective study in man has provided most of the needed answers.(12) Ward et al demonstrated that prophylactic barbiturates in head trauma (i.e., patients were randomized without regard to initial ICP levels) administered for at least 72 hours had no influence whatsoever on outcome (the only significant difference was a higher incidence of hypotension in the treated groups). Although this was not an ICP study per se it is interesting to note that there were no differences between the two groups in the mean ICP, the incidence and magnitude of episodic increases in ICP, or the incidence of uncontrolled ICP. The results at least suggest that although barbiturate therapy offers an alternative approach to controlling ICP, it is no better than other aggressive forms of therapy (hyperosmotic agents and hyperventilation). Certainly the results support the conclusion that barbiturates do not offer any unusual "protective" effect in head trauma.

From a cerebral metabolic standpoint isoflurane at concentrations of 2 MAC should provide the same potential for protection as high dose barbiturate therapy. At 2 MAC isoflurane produces an isoelectric EEG and in dogs the cerebral metabolic profile appears to be identical to that encountered with barbiturate induced EEG isoelectricity.(13) Also in a dog model of acute global ischemia isoflurane provides for a degree of protection similar to that seen with barbiturates.(14) When profound hypotension (MAP < 40 mmHg) is induced in dogs with isoflurane for 1 hour the cerebral metabolic profile is normal whereas a similar level of hypotension induced by trimethaphan, nitroprusside, or halothane is associated with significant cerebral metabolic perturbations.(15) In man during carotid endarterectomy the critical

CBF during carotid occlusion (i.e., the CBF below which ischemic EEG changes occur) is significantly reduced to 8-10 $ml \cdot 100g^{-1} \cdot min^{-1}$ with isoflurane anesthesia as compared with that seen during halothane or enflurane anesthesia (18-20 $ml \cdot 100g^{-1} \cdot min^{-1}$).[16] Presumably this is again explained by greater cerebral metabolic suppression with isoflurane.

A potential major differences between barbiturates and isoflurane is that the latter is a modest cerebral vasodilator while barbiturates are associated with decreased CBF (in parallel with the decrease in $CMRO_2$). This suggests the possibility that in focal ischemia isoflurane may differ from barbiturates (because of a possible intracerebral steal). Todd et al have reported in a primate model of transient (6 hours) focal ischemia (produced by middle cerebral artery occlusion) that isoflurane anesthetized animals had a significantly worse outcome than thiopental anesthetized animals in terms of frequency and size of infarcts and nearly significant differences were observed in terms of neurologic deficits on day 7 post ischemia ($p = 0.06$).[17] Although highly suggestive that isoflurane offers no protection in focal ischemia (despite the lower critical CBF in man?) there are two problems with the Todd et al study: 1) all of the thiopental treated animals received high dose nitroprusside for over 6 hours during and after ischemia while all of the isoflurane animals received phenylephrine during this period, and 2) despite these drug differences mean arterial pressure was significantly greater in the thiopental treated animals throughout the period of ischemia (approximately 85 vs 105 mmHg). The effects of these drug and pefusion pressure differences on the outcome are major unknowns and at this time no definitive conclusions are possible regarding the effects of isoflurane in focal ischemia.

Another group of drugs that may offer beneficial effects during or after cerebral ischemia are certain calcium entry blockers which appear to have a prediliction for cerebral as opposed to systemic vascular smooth muscle. Two such drugs which show promise in animal models are nimodipine and lidoflazine. In man nimodipine has been reported to significantly reduce the deleterious effects of cerebral vasospasm in patients suffering from subarachnoid hemorrhage.[18]

In the event of complete global ischemia (cardiac arrest) reperfusion is characterized by an immediate reactive hyperemia followed within 20-30 minutes by a delayed post ischemic hypoperfusion state.[19] It has been postulated that the latter contributes to the ultimate neurologic outcome. In animals nimodipine given either before or after the ischemic period will either prevent or attenuate this hypoperfusion state.[20,21] In a primate study nimodipine given after 17 minutes of complete ischemia significantly improved both the neurologic outcome and the histopathologic effects of the ischemic episode.(22) It is tempting to conclude that the improved outcome is accounted for by the improved blood flow. However, lidoflazine has no effect on post global ischemic CBF but may nonetheless improve outcome.(23) The latter studies of outcome are somewhat conflicting(24,25) and no primate studies have yet been reported. Should the latter demonstrate unequivocally improved outcome a mechanism other than improved CBF must be invoked, while the presumed mechanism for improved outcome with nimodipine might be questioned.

There have been numerous other pharmacologic interventions suggested or tested for possible brain "protection". These include phenytoin, naloxone, mannitol, steroids, various anesthetics (other than barbiturates and isoflurane) and compounds which might attenuate damage from free oxygen radicals during the post ischemic phase. The latter includes the iron chelator, deferoxamine, which by binding available iron should partially block free radical formation. However, in a dog model of complete cerebral ischemia, pretreatment with deferoxamine did not alter neurologic outcome.(26) Similarly the enzymes catalase and super oxide dismutase should minimize free radical damage but again failed to alter neurologic outcome in the same dog model.(27)

An important determinant of outcome following cerebral ischemia appears to be the blood (and brain) glucose levels at the time of the ischemia. Even modest increases in glucose as produced by the pre ischemic infusion of a 5% dextrose solution (10-15 ml/kg) has been shown in primates to significantly aggravate neurologic outcome.(28) In that study mean pre ischemic glucose was 180 mg/dl vs 140 mg/dl in animals not given a dextrose solution. Clinically it would seem prudent to avoid intraoperative infusion of glucose containing solutions in patients who might experience a transient period of cerebral ischemia (e.g., intracranial and cerebrovascular procedures).

REFERENCES

1. Abramson, N.S. N. Engl. J. Med. 314:397-403, 1986.

2. Steen, P.A., Milde J.D. and Michenfelder J.D. Ann. Neurol. 5:343-349, 1979.

3. Todd, M.M, Chadwick, H.S., Shapiro, H.M., Dunlap, M.J., Marshall, L.F. and Dueck R. Anesthesiology 57:76-86, 1982.

4. Gisvold, S.E., Safar, P., Hendricks, H.H.L., Rao, G., Moossy, G. and Alexander H. Anesthesiology 60:88-96, 1984.

5. Smith, A.L., Hoff, J.T., Nielsen, S.L. and Larson, C.P. Stroke 5:127, 1974.

6. Michenfelder, J.D. and Milde J.H. Stroke 6:405-410, 1975.

7. Michenfelder, J.D., Milde J.H. and Sundt, T.M., Jr. Arch. Neurol. 33:345-350, 1976.

8. Nussmeier, N.A., Arlund, C. and Slogoff S. Anesthesiology 64:171-174, 1986.

9. Ehrenhaft, J.L., Claman, M.A., Layton, J.M. and Zimmerman, G.R. J. Thorac. Cardiovasc. Surg. 42:514-526, 1961.

10. Gilman, S. N. Engl. J. Med. 272:489-498, 1965.

11. Tufo, H.M., Ostfeld, A.M. and Shekelle, R. J.A.M.A. 212:1333-1340, 1970.

12. Ward, J.D., Becker, D.P., Miller, D.J., Choy, S.C., Marmarou, A., Wood, C., Newlon, P.G. and Keenan, R. Neurosurg. 62:383-388, 1985.

13. Newberg, L.A., Milde, J.H. and Michenfelder, J.D. Anesthesiology 59:23-28, 1983.

14. Newberg, L.A. and Michenfelder, J.D. Anesthesiology 59:29-35, 1983.

15. Newberg, L.A., Milde, J.H. and Michenfelder, J.D. Anesthesiology 60:541-546, 1984.

16. Casement, B., Messick, J., Milde L, et. al. Anesthesiology 63:A406, 1985.

17. Todd, M.M., Hehls, D.G., Drummond, J.C., et. al. Anesthesiology 63:A412, 1985.

18. Allen, G.S., Ahn, H.S., Preziosi, T.J., et. al. N. Engl. J. Med. 308:619-624, 1983.

19. Steen, P.A., Milde, J.H. and Michenfelder, J.D. J. Neurochem. 31:1317-1324, 1978.

20. Steen, P.A., Newberg, L.A., Milde, J.H. and Michenfelder, J.D. J. Cereb. Blood Flow Metab. 3:38-43, 1983.

21. Steen, P.A., Newberg, L.A., Milde, J.H. and Michenfelder, J.D. J. Cereb. Blood Flow Metab. 4:82-87, 1984.

22. Steen, P.A., Gisvold, S.E., Milde, J.H., Newberg, L.A., Scheithauer, B.W., Lanier, W.L. and Michenfelder, J.D. Anesthesiology 62:406-414, 1985.

23. Fleischer, J.E., Lanier, W.L. and Michenfelder, J.D. In preparation.
24. Vaagenes, P., Cantadore, R, Safar, P., Moossy, J., Rao, G., Diven, W., Alexander, H. and Stezoski, W. Crit. Care Med. 12:846-855, 1984.
25. Vaagenes, P., Cantadore, R., Safar, P. and Alexander, H. Anesthesiology 59:A100, 1983.
26. Fleischer, J.E. and Michenfelder, J.D. In preparation.
27. Steen, P.A. and Michenfelder, J.D. In preparation.
28. Lanier, W.L., Stangland, K.J., Scheithauer, B.W., et. al. Anesthesiology 63:A110, 1985.

DELIBERATE HYPOTENSION

E.D. MILLER, JR.

In the late 1940's and the early 1950's a great deal of research concerning the pharmacology of muscle relaxants and related compounds was begun. It was at this time it was discovered that some agents, namely hexamathonium, had a profound effect on the blood pressure, while other compounds of a similar series had more effect on neuromuscular blocking. Shortly after this time, Enderby used one such compound in this series to produce controlled hypotension in patients (1). Since that time, there have been strong advocates both for and against methods to lower blood pressure electively. The terms, "controlled hypotension," "induced hypotension," "deliberate hypotension," and "hypotensive anesthesia" have all been applied, but for this discussion the term, "deliberate hypotension," will be used. The main purpose of deliberate hypotension is to decrease blood loss, and thereby decrease the need for blood transfusion and/or improve operating conditions at the surgical site. The latter, namely, improved visibility for the surgeon, is more difficult to quantitate but is certainly a strong argument in favor of its use.

EFFECT OF HYPOTENSION ON BLOOD LOSS

The best documentation that decreasing blood pressure decreases blood loss appears in studies done on patients undergoing major orthopedic procedures. In several of the studies that have recently been reported, it has been well demonstrated that blood loss can be reduced to approximately 50% of that seen in patients who do not have their blood pressure decreased. In most of the studies done, mean blood pressure has been decreased to 50-60 mmHg. However, it should be pointed out that these are not magic numbers and that, in some instances, blood loss will continue even though the blood pressure has been decreased to this level. Part of this difficulty in decreasing blood loss may be due to improper positioning of the patient so that venous drainage is not adequate. Another important aspect is that ventilation be controlled so that high levels of carbon dioxide do not persist, which is also known to cause stimulation of the sympathetic nervous system. The cause of the decreased blood loss during deliberate hypotension is related to the decrease in mean arterial pressure and not to decreased cardiac output. This has been well documented by Sivarajan and co-workers who studied 20 healthy subjects undergoing bilateral sagittal osteotomies of the mandible. They used either trimethaphan or sodium nitroprusside to lower blood pressure and found that blood loss was similar in both groups even though cardiac output was markedly different in the two drug treatments.

METHODS TO ACHIEVE DELIBERATE HYPOTENSION

A variety of techniques to produce deliberate hypotension has been devised. The earliest technique to reduce arterial pressure was controlled hemorrhage through an arteriotomy. However, it would seem that this is too dangerous a technique since cardiac output is markedly impaired and, therefore, organ infusion may also be impaired before a significant decrease in mean arterial pressure occurs.

The use of spinal anesthesia or epidural anesthesia would also be an acceptable way to produce hypotension. Problems with this technique, however, range from the inability to reverse the effects quickly to a lesser degree of control than one could achieve by other means.

Certainly the use of inhalation agents would be another way to produce hypotension. The earliest agent that was used was halothane which at first was thought to be an ideal agent because of vasodilatation. However, the studies by Prys-Roberts and co-workers showed that the effects of profound hypotension by halothane were due to a significant decrease in cardiac output without much change on peripheral vascular resistance. It was during this study that one patient suffered a cardiac arrest while ventilated with 2% halothane and oxygen, and there was considerable difficulty in resuscitating this patient (2). Recently, with the introduction of isoflurane there have been reports that this may be an acceptable way to produce hypotension since the main effect of isoflurane is to decrease peripheral resistance and allow cardiac output to remain near normal levels.

While the above techniques will achieve a blood pressure in the hypotensive range, most would agree that the use of intravenous agents is one of the more controllable methods to produce hypotension. The agents that are available range from sodium nitroprusside, nitroglycerin, and trimethaphan to some newer agents such as adenosine, hydralazine, prostaglandin E1, and labetalol. Each of these agents is able to produce hypotension but through different mechanisms. Sodium nitroprusside, probably the most commonly used agent, decreases blood pressure by decreasing arterial peripheral resistance with some effects on the venous side of the circulation. Intravenous nitroglycerin, on the other hand, has a predominant effect on the venous side of the circulation and at higher doses affects the arterial circulation as well. Nitroprusside is noted to have a greater degree of flexibility than intravenous nitroglycerin and is the preferred agent in many cases. Trimethaphan, a ganglionic blocker, has been used for a long time to control blood pressure. Trimethaphan produces a decrease in both arteriolar and venous tone, and autonomic reflexes are blocked. Other agents have also been used to decrease blood pressure through a direct effect on the arterials. Hydralazine, for instance, is able to lower mean arterial blood pressure with intravenous doses but is not quite as controllable as an intravenous infusion where the effect can be terminated rapidly. The newer agents such as adenosine and ATP may prove to be beneficial in the future. A side effect of ATP and adenosine is complete heart block in some patients, which may prevent its use. Labetalol, a combined alpha- and beta-receptor antagonist, has some attractive features to it. Not only does it block alpha receptors and therefore decrease blood pressure by this means, but the reflex increase in heart rate when the blood pressure decreases would be prevented by the simultaneous blocking of the beta-receptors. When this drug becomes available in the United States, it will have interesting therapeutic implications.

INFLUENCE OF HYPOTENSION ON ORGAN FUNCTION

In order for hypotension to be a realistic therapeutic intervention it must be demonstrated that periods of hypotension are not detrimental to the various organs of the body. Multiple studies have been done attempting to answer this question. Certainly data suggest that when one lowers blood pressure with any of the agents previously mentioned, there are marked decreases in blood flow to both muscle and skin. It is crucial that these two beds have such a response. If they did not, then blood loss could not be minimized. The next organ that is of prime importance whenever deliberate hypotension is used is the brain. Adequacy of cerebral perfusion during induced hypotension has been studied by a variety of techniques. Many of these techniques, although relatively crude tools to measure cerebral function, show that deliberate hypotension does not produce permanent changes in cerebral function. However, the data examining the various modes of inducing hypotension have shown conflicting results. The current rationale for the safe lower limit of mean arterial pressure of 50-55 mmHg in normothermic patients is based on the concept that the lower limit of autoregulation for cerebral blood flow is at this range. Michenfelder and Theye saw clear neurologic deficits in two of the five dogs anesthetized with nitrous oxide and subjected to one hour of hypotension at a mean pressure of 40 mmHg by trimethaphan (3). However, Dong and associates demonstrated that there was a poor correlation between EEG and brain function when dogs were subjected to profound hypotension (4). In their study, a mean arterial pressure between 12 and 25 mmHg for one hour was achieved with trimethaphan. These investigators thought that organs other than the brain were at a higher degree of risk when such severe degrees of hypotension were used.

A wealth of information is available comparing the effects of nitroprusside, nitroglycerin, and trimethaphan when used to control blood pressure intraoperatively. For years a history of coronary artery disease has been a contraindication for deliberate hypotension. Some patients, such as those undergoing clipping of a cerebral aneurysm, may require hypotension to help in the surgical procedure. These same patients may also have underlying coronary artery disease, and therefore knowledge concerning the use of these agents during deliberate hypotension is important. Recently, Hickey and co-workers have examined the effects of induced hypotension in a dog model with single coronary artery stenosis (5). Hypotension was induced with trimethaphan, halothane, or sodium nitroprusside to a mean arterial pressure of 50 mmHg. Their data show that, with a critical stenosis, hypotension resulted in reduced regional myocardial blood flow. However, myocardial ischemia was not found. There was continued lactate extraction, no changes in ST segments, and no redistribution of transmural blood flow. It should be noted that this was done in a dog model and the stenosis involved only one vessel which is not the common clinical finding. It does suggest that our concerns about deliberate hypotension in patients with coronary artery disease may not be as justified as we once thought.

The effects of deliberate hypotension on pulmonary circulation have been studied for some time. It had been thought that with controlled hypotension there would be an increase in the physiologic deadspace. However, when examined critically, it was found that if cardiac output was maintained at the pre-hypotensive level, no increase in deadspace was found. Secondly, oxygenation during deliberate hypotension may be altered. Most workers have demonstrated that with a marked decrease in arterial blood pressure there is a decrease in oxygenation as well, and this should be considered when using such a technique. The other effects of hypotensive agents on pulmonary function are minimal.

The kidneys have also been an area of great concern whenever hypotensive agents have been used. Most data suggest that, while renal blood flow is decreased during hypotensive anesthesia, no untoward effects are able to be demonstrated. It would appear, from the data from a variety of investigators, that induced hypotension for short periods of time does not have a detrimental effect on the kidneys.

The splanchnic circulation is one of the more difficult areas to evaluate. Since the portal circulation has no significant autoregulation and hepatic regulation is minimal, it is possible that the liver could be severely damaged during periods of deliberate hypotension. This appears to be true only when severe degrees of hypotension are employed; but when the normal 50-65 mmHg mean arterial pressure is used as the end point, there seems to be little change in the liver function test.

CLINICAL USE OF CONTROLLED HYPOTENSION

The preceding discussion illustrates the many facets which are involved when one considers the use of deliberate hypotension. The concern of the anesthesiologist should be directed not only at drug selection but also at the type of surgery, length of procedure, need to decrease blood loss, and patient suitability.

There are many indications for the use of deliberate hypotension. Major uses include neurosurgical procedures, large orthopedic procedures, complicated back surgery, surgery on large tumors, surgery of the head and neck, and a variety of plastic surgical procedures. The contraindications in the use of hypotension have relaxed over the years with better drugs, better monitoring, and more experience with the technique, which has allowed more patients to benefit from this than previously. The major consideration in deciding if a patient is a suitable candidate for deliberate hypotension is knowledge of the suitability of the patient for such a technique. A history of cerebral vascular disease, renal dysfunction, liver dysfunction, or severe peripheral claudication would suggest that the patient may be less than likely to have good organ perfusion during periods of hypotension. Similarly, patients with hypovolemia or severe anemia would not be suitable candidates since their reserve is markedly altered already.

The decision to use deliberate hypotension in a patient with long-standing hypertension is difficult. Recent data suggest that the treatment of hypertension restores the autoregulatory process of the brain, but whether this data can be applied to man is difficult to judge. Similarly a history of a myocardial infarction several years previously does not necessarily exclude the patient, but one must weigh the benefit/risk ratio.

MONITORING DURING DELIBERATE HYPOTENSION

Arterial blood pressure measurement on a beat-to-beat basis seems justified in patients whose blood pressure will be lowered significantly.

Some might suggest that the automatic noninvasive blood pressure apparatus would be adequate if severe degrees of hypotension are not to be employed. EKG monitoring and temperature monitoring should also be routine. If large blood losses are anticipated, a central venous catheter or a pulmonary artery catheter should be selected depending on the patient. In prolonged procedures measurement of urinary output is also necessary. Other measurements of electrolyte, blood gas analysis, and hematocrit throughout the case should be routine. The measurement of central venous oxygen prior to induced hypotension would be helpful in patients receiving sodium nitroprusside since a rise in oxygen might suggest cyanide toxicity. Other monitors that could be used include evoked potentials, EEG, and tissue pH, but these need further evaluation before they become routine monitors.

COMPLICATIONS

As in much of our practice, it is difficult to define precisely the incident of complications that occur when deliberate hypotension is used. In a very large series, looking at 9,000 patients, Enderby thought that only 0.055% of the deaths could be related to anesthesia and hypotension. Nonfatal complications probably are more common, however. Complications such as dizziness, prolonged awakening, cerebral thrombosis, blurred vision, and blindness seem to be related to the central nervous system. However, bleeding into the operative site, postoperative anuria or oliguria, and persistent hypotension have also been listed. In the present day it is extremely difficult to judge precisely the morbidity and mortality associated with deliberate hypotension. From the data available, hypotension to 50-60 mmHg in the young, well-monitored patient appears to be safe. Unfortunately, many of the patients in whom deliberate hypotension may be of advantage have underlying organ dysfunction which cannot be easily appreciated by routine examination. It is imperative, therefore, that in all patients in whom deliberate hypotension is considered, a thorough and complete examination of the individual be done prior to the time of operation. Deliberate hypotension should not be decided upon in the operating room without careful thought to the potential complications.

SUMMARY

Deliberate hypotension is an effective means to decrease blood loss and provide a surgical field that ensures better visibility of vital structures. Numerous techniques and agents have been developed to lower blood pressure. The mode of action in these agents is different and results in complex alterations in reflexes and subsequent changes in blood flow to various organs. Deliberate hypotension is not without risk, however, and the advantages and disadvantages need to be considered. The intelligent use of deliberate hypotension has distinct advantages for certain procedures and it may insure surgical success. Deliberate hypotension should be a technique that we are able to offer our surgical colleagues in order to provide the best in anesthesia care to surgical patients.

REFERENCES

1. Enderby, G.E.H. Lancet 1:1145, 1950.

2. Prys-Roberts, C,, Lloyd, J.W., Fisher, A., Kerr, J.H., and Patterson, T.J. Br J Anaesth 46:105, 1974.

3. Michenfelder, J.D. and Theye, R.A. Anesthesiology 46:188, 1977.

4. Dong, W.K., Bledsoe, S.W., Eng, D.Y., Heavner, J.E., Shaw, C.M., Hornbein, T.F., and Anderson, J.L. Anesthesiology 58:61, 1983.

5. Hickey, R.F., Verrier, E.D., Baer, R.W., Vlahakes, C.J., Fein, G. and Hoffman, J.I.E. Anesthesiology 59:226, 1983.

ANAESTHETIC MANAGEMENT OF PULMONARY THROMBOENDARTERECTOMY

Simon de Lange, M.D.

Acute pulmonary embolism is a common complication which often afflicts hospitalized patients after trauma and surgery. The overall incidence in both medical and surgical patients is approximately 20 per 1000 hospital admissions with a mortality rate of about 25 % of this figure (1). Usually medical treatment with anticoagulants and thrombolytic therapy resolves the disease process but occasionally surgical intervention is required when medical treatment has failed and a massive pulmonary embolism precipitates cardio-respiratory arrest. However, the surgical results of acute pulmonary embolectomy have been unimpressive since Trendelenberg proposed this heroic procedure in 1908; the first survivor was only reported in 1924 (2). In fact by 1961 when the first successful pulmonary embolectomy was performed with the aid of cardiopulmonary bypass, only 22 survivors of the Trendelenberg procedure were recorded in the literature - a mortality rate greater than 95 % (3).

A recent study showed that cardiopulmonary bypass, especially if this was a portable facility, afforded a somewhat better chance of survival in moribund patients with acute, massive pulmonary embolism; even then half of the operated patients died (2). Transvenous removal of emboli by vacuum-cup catheter technique has been recommended as an alternative method of effectively (and less traumatically) managing acute major pulmonary embolism especially in hospitals that do not have the capability of cardiopulmonary bypass (4).

In the acute attack these clots may be scooped or sucked out of the pulmonary arteries but if they remain and fibrinolysis does not occur they become organised and adhere to the vessel wall so that removal will need careful dissection (pulmonary thromboendarterectomy).

CHRONIC PULMONARY EMBOLISM

Fortunately after acute pulmonary embolism the circulation usually re-establishes itself in the compromised pulmonary arteries (5). Resolution of emboli occurs naturally by fibrinolysis which takes about 7-10 days. Medical therapy with heparin and streptokinase can promote this process and reduce the overall mortality rate by about 8 % (1).

If pulmonary embolism remains undiagnosed, and therefore untreated, or if medical treatment has been inadequate, there is an increased risk of repeated emboli. In a small but definite group of patients the emboli do not resolve, possibly because they were already partially organized before embolization (6). The continued presence of emboli in the pulmonary arteries three months after the first acute episode is defined as chronic pulmonary embolism. The persisting clots become fibrotic and firmly adherant to the arterial wall (7). Further embolization exacerbates the disease process and results in pulmonary hypertension with cor pulmonale, tricuspid valve insufficiency and eventually death (8).

Medical management has been directed at the treatment of pulmonary hypertension and inhibiting the formation of further emboli by anticoagulant therapy. Pulmonary vasodilatation had not been achieved with nifedipine, prazozine or catopril (9). Neither thrombolytic therapy with streptokinase nor anticoagulant therapy with heparin or phenprocoumon have afforded symptomatic relief (9, 10).

PULMONARY THROMBOENDARTERECTOMY

The surgical approach offers some hope against a lingering, asphyxial death. The first successful embolectomy (endarterectomy) for chronic pulmonary embolism was reported in 1958 (11). Since then over 50 cases have been described with about a 75 % operative survival rate. In many of these patients there was good relief of symptoms, some returning to normal work, but in a few there was little change (6-12).

Indications for surgery in the reported cases have been:

1. Severe dyspnoea at rest or with minimal exertion, NYHA functional class III or IV (6, 12).
2. Pulmonary hypertension, systolic pressure above 50 mmHg, increased pulmonary vascular resistance with a normal capillary wedge pressure (6, 9, 10, 12).

3. Angiographic demonstration of more than 50 % occlusion in the lobar arteries or central to the lobar arteries (6, 10, 12).

SURGICAL MANAGEMENT

A median sternotomy or a lateral thoracotomy approach of the - pulmonary arteries may be used (6-12). However, the central approach is currently favoured by several authors since division of the pericardium bilaterally to the pulmonary arteries with retraction of the phrenic nerves permits direct exposure of the lobar arteries (6, 9, 12). Usually extracorporeal circulatory support is necessary.

Whilst on full cardiopulmonary bypass considerable backflow bleeding has occured in many cases during endarterectomy and has been interpreted as a highly favourable sign that the artery will subsequently remain patent (6, 7). Extensive anastomoses are formed between the bronchial arteries and the pulmonary circulation at precapillary level so that the smaller vessels remain patent and thus making thromboendarterectomy a feasible operation even after years of pulmonary artery obstruction (7). However, backflow bleeding has hampered dissection so that deep hypothermia and circulatory arrest have been used to facilitate surgery (6, 9, 12). Careful internal dissection of the pulmonary arteries has freed cylinders of intima or casts which embody organised thrombi some of which have been found to be of different ages and stages of fibrosis (6, 9, 12).

Over 95 % of pulmonary emboli originate in the deep veins of the legs and pelvis, the femoral and iliac veins (13). To avoid further embolization inferior vena caval interruption is also done during the operation especially if there is continued evidence of thrombophlebitis (9, 10).

ANAESTHETIC MANAGEMENT

Monitoring Standard monitoring should be done with ECG, radial artery and thermodilution pulmonary artery catheters. There exists some controversy about placement of a pulmonary artery catheter for this procedure because of concern that it might contribute to a postoperative recurrence of pulmonary artery thrombosis (12). However there are no reports at present which justify this concern (10).

The tip of the catheter is manipulated so that it lies in the proximal part of the pulmonary artery and thus does not hamper surgery. Use of a sterile external sleeve around the catheter permits repositioning when necessary. It is essential that cardiac output and pulmonary artery pressures are measured during and after these operations since low output syndrome often occurs with a high pulmonary vascular resistance so that judicious titration of inotropes and vasodilation therapy is required to improve cardiac function. The pulmonary artery catheter is removed within 48 hours of placement if possible to reduce risk of infection.

Inotropic support These patients have chronic cor pulmonale which can eventually also compromize left ventricular function (14). Thus, right-sided failure secondary to pulmonary hypertension is present and left-sided failure may be incipient and precipitated during the stress of anaesthesia and surgery. Dobutamine has been recommended as a suitable inotrope under these conditions (10). This is also our experience but occasionally an additional infusion of cathecholamines (adrenaline and isoprenaline) has been required to maintain a cardiac index above 2.0 after cardiopulmonary bypass.

Vasodilator therapy has been attempted in order to reduce the high pulmonary vascular resistance which may limit cardiac output in this disease. Hydralazine, nifedipine, prazozine and catopril caused systemic hypotension and reflex tachycardia but have had no beneficial effect on pulmonary artery pressure or cardiac output (9, 15). However nitroglycerine, when used in treating pulmonary hypertension, has been shown to significantly decrease pulmonary vascular resistance in a dosage that did not result in systemic hypotension. But the reduction in right-sided afterload allowed a significant increase in cardiac output; under similar conditions sodium nitroprusside had no significant effect on pulmonary vascular resistance or cardiac output (16). We routinely use a nitroglycerine infusion (0,25 - 0,5 mcg/kg/min) as vasodilator therapy both during surgery and in the ICU.

Anaesthetic technique We premedicate these extremely ill and hypoxic patients with lorazepam 0,03 - 0,04 mg/kg per os but avoid the respiratory depressant action of opioids preoperatively. If patients are taking chronic, long-acting nitrate therapy it is also given with the premedication.

Nitrous oxide is not used since it may increase pulmonary vascular resistance (17). Volatile inhalational agents can cause myocardial depression and can also inhibit hypoxic pulmonary vasoconstriction. These patients already have an increased ventilation - perfusion mismatch with chronic hypoxaemia and impaired cardiac function, so volatile agents are also avoided.

Since 1982 we have performed about two pulmonary thromboendarterectomies per year in our clinic and have found high dose fentanyl (75-100 mcg/kg) a very suitable anaesthetic technique. Combined with parcuronium as muscle relaxant it affords cardiovascular stability and allows a high inspired oxygen concentration in these severely hypoxic patients. Furthermore, fentanyl anaesthesia is considered not to increase pulmonary vascular resistance and it may even promote pulmonary blood flow. In contrast to inhalational anaesthetic agents, intravenous agents do not affect the hypoxic pulmonary vasoconstrictor reflex (18). Thus, with fentanyl anaesthesia the ventilation-perfusion mismatch, which may be substantial in these patients is not increased. We find that these patients all develop reperfusion pulmonary oedema in the desobstructed areas of lung after cardiopulmonary bypass so that postoperative ventilatory support is necessary which is also facilitated by the high dose fentanyl technique.

Fentanyl anaesthesia can inhibit the low levels of sympathetic activity which is required to maintain venous tone. A high systemic venous tone is necessary to maintain the venous return required to fill a dilated and poorly compliant ventricle (19). We find that a systemic vasopressor may be required together with a fluid load to maintain venous return during induction with fentanyl. Ketamine centrally stimulates the release of endogenous cathecholamines as well as providing dissociative anaesthesia. A combined ketamine (0,5-1,0 mg/kg) and fentanyl induction has also afforded us stable cardiovascular condition in these poor risk cases.

We do not use a double-lumen endobronchial intubation technique routinely in our anaesthetic management since the median sternotomy approach is preferred in our clinic and these tubes can cause bronchial trauma. They are also uncomfortable for the patient in the ICU. We would employ endobroncial intubation if a lateral thoractomy approach were to be used or if there had been a recent episode of haemoptysis (10, 12). We are also prepared to reintubate with a double-lumen endobronchial tube if reperfusion lung oedema was unilateral profuse and haemorrhagic as repor-

110

ted inone patient, and where differential pulmonary ventilation was indicated (12).

POSTOPERATIVE COMPLICATIONS

Reperfusion pulmonary oedema occurs in the desobstructed lung fields after cardiopulmonary bypass and is thought to be caused by an increased capillary permeability (10, 12). Postoperative ventilatory support is necessary for 48 hours or even longer whilst the oedema subsides with the aid of diuretics (12). Judicious use of PEEP may be needed during this period to attain an acceptable arterial oxygen tension. Rarely respiratory distress syndrome develops or there is phrenic nerve injury and ventilation for longer periods may be required (10, 12).

Other complications recorded in the literature are haemorrhage with haemoptysis, infarction of the lung due to migration of an embolus, reocclusion of the pulmonary arteries, infections, pyopneumothorax and haematothorax (6-12).

Cardiac failure, especially right heart failure, may occur postoperatively and may need prolonged inotropic support.

Fortunately, in most patients who have undergone pulmonary thrombo-endarterectomy there was an improvement in their cardio-pulmonary status. In some patients, who had been severely handicapped, the improvement was so great that they could return to a normal life.

1. Sasahara AA, Sharma GVRK, Barsamian EM, Schoolman M, Cella G: Pulmonary thromboembolism. Diagnosis and treatment. JAMA 249: 2945-2950, 1983.

2. Mattox KL, Feldtman RW, Beall AC Jr, De Bakey ME: Pulmonary embolectomy for acute massive pulmonary embolism. Ann Surg 195: 726-731 1982.

3. Cooley DA, Beall AC Jr, Alexander JK: Acute massive pulmonary embolism: successful surgical treatment using temporary cardiopulmonary bypass. JAMA 177: 283-286, 1961.

4. Stewart JR, Greenfield LJ: Transvenous venacaval filtration and pulmonary embolectomy. Surg Clin N Am 62: 411-430, 1982.

5. Dalen JE, Alpert JS: Natural history of pulmonary embolism. Prog Cardiovasc Dis 17: 259-270, 1975.

6. Daily PO, Johnston GG, Simmons CJ, Moser KM: Surgical management of chronic pulmonary embolism. Surgical treatment and late results. J Thorac Cardiovasc Surg 79: 523-531, 1980.

7. Sabiston DC Jr, Wolfe WG, Oldham HN Jr, Wechsler AS, Crawford FA Jr, Jones KW, Jones RH: Surgical management of chronic pulmonary embolism Ann Surg 185: 699-712, 1977.

8. Moser KM, Houk VN, Jones RC, Hufnagel CC: Chronic, massive thrombotic obstruction of the pulmonary arteries. Analysis of four operated cases. Circulation 32: 377-385, 1965.

9. Drost H, Kolff J, Huysmans HA, Buis B: Geslaagde tromboendarteriëctomie bij een patiënte met chronische longembolie. Ned Tijdschr Geneeskd 127: 2091-2094, 1983.

10. Brown DL, Bodary AK, Kirby RR: Anesthetic management of pulmonary thromboendarterectomy. Anesthesiology 61: 197-200, 1984.

11. Allison PR, Dunhill MS, Marshall R: Pulmonary embolism. Thorax 15: 273-279, 1960.

12. Utley JR, Spragg RG, Long WB, Moser KM: Pulmonary endarterectomy for chronic thromboembolic obstruction: Recent surgical experience. Surgery 92: 1096-1102, 1982.

13. Moser KM: Pulmonary embolism. Am Rev Respir Dis 115: 829-852, 1977.

14. Frank MJ, Weiss AB, Moschos CB, Levinson GE: Left ventricular function, metabolism and blood flow in chronic cor pulmonale. Circulation 47: 798-806, 1973.

15. Packer M, Greenberg B, Massie B, Dash H: Deleterious effects of hydralazine in patients with pulmonary hypertension. N Engl J Med 306: 1326-1331, 1982.

16. Rosenthal MH, Pearl RG, Schroeder JS, Ashton JPA: Nitroglycerin versus nitroprusside in pulmonary hypertension. Anesthesiology 55: A79, 1981.

17. Hilgenberg JC, McCammon RL, Stoelting RK: Pulmonary and systemic vascular responses to nitrous oxide in patients with stenosis and pulmonary hypertension. Anesth. Analg. 59: 323-326, 1980.

18. Bjertnaes LJ: Hypoxia-induced vasoconstriction in isolated perfused lungs exposed to injectable or inhalational anaesthetics. Acta Anaesthesiol. Scand. 21: 133-147, 1977.

19. Gaffney TE, Braunwald E: Importance of the adrenergic nervous system in support of circulatory function in patients with congestive heart failure. Am J Med 34: 320-324, 1963.

ANESTHESIA FOR ADULT CARDIAC SURGERY

J. ARENS

Adult cardiac surgery is the largest surgical service in many hospitals and open heart surgery has almost become commonplace. Every anesthesiologist needs to understand the basic anesthetic principles of cardiovascular anesthesia, not only for the safe management of these patients, but for the management of cardiac patients presenting for non-cardiac surgery.

Coronary artery bypass grafting (CABG) for coronary artery disease continues to be the most prevalent procedure in adult cardiac surgery. The preoperative evaluation of these patients is a subject of great debate. Patients undergoing CABG will have had a cardiac catheterization with the extent and site of coronary disease delineated. Areas of myocardial wall dyskinesia are identified and frequently the ejection fraction is calculated. Left ventricular end diastolic pressure is recorded as well as the pulmonary artery (PA) pressures. These data are important to the anesthesiologist for many reasons. For example, patients with right coronary lesions frequently have sinus bradycardia or nodal rhythms, and the presence of significant congestive heart failure is a predictor of mortality. It is important to recognize that the data collected during cardiac catheterization represents dynamic, not static, data. Nevertheless, major anesthetic decisions continue to be based upon single pressures, measured at one point in time, in the cath lab.

The CASS study (a multicenter study) has been an ongoing attempt to reveal predictors of outcome for patients receiving CABG. These data indicated that the factors which had the most adverse influence on mortality included left main coronary disease, mitral regurgitation, congestive failure, myocardial dyskinesia, chronic hypertension, age, sex, ejection fraction and LVEDP (1). Recently, ischemia before bypass, cross-clamp time, quality of anastomoses and finesse of the anesthesiologist have been shown to influence the incidence of perioperative myocardial infarction (2). The anesthesiologist who had the greatest incidence of perioperative myocardial infarctions also had the highest incidence of perioperative tachycardia which is a major determinant of myocardial oxygen economics. Anesthesia technique, therefore, may be more important than which agents are administered. The quality of anastomoses is also influenced by the extent of the patient's coronary artery disease and the aptitude of the surgeon.

The preoperative evaluation of the adult cardiac patient includes a knowledge of drug therapy such as beta blockade, calcium channel blockers, anti-hypertensive drugs, anti-arrhythmics, etc. Dogmatic statements about perioperative drug therapy are often more anecdotal than factual. However, the preoperative period is not the time to adjust, reduce, or withdraw a patient from chronic drug therapy which has achieved hemodynamic stability. Beta blockers should not be withdrawn prior to surgery. In general, it is agreed that drugs should be continued throughout the perioperative period.

Concepts about the coronary circulation and its pathology continues its dynamic evolution. A rebirth of internal mammary artery - coronary artery anastomoses has occurred. The long term patency rate of the arterial-arterial anastomoses has been higher than that of the venous to arterial. Thus, IMA's tend to be done in younger patients. The site of arterial line placement, site of CVP (Swan-Ganz) placement, degree of postop pain, and severity of ventilatory dysfunction will be influenced by IMA surgery. Coronary spasm has become the disease of the 80's especially with the advent of calcium channel blockers (3). This phenomenon was originally described by Osler in 1910 and popularized by Prinzmetal in 1959. Coronary spasm can occur in normal as well as in atherosclerotic coronary arteries. Classically, ST segment elevation occurs over the site corresponding to the artery in spasm. In addition, left ventricular dysfunction occurs with a decrease in cardiac output and an increase in pulmonary artery occluded pressure. Nitroglycerine may be effective; however, sublingual nifedipine often produces dramatic improvement. Beta blockers alone may not be effective agents and in fact may exacerbate the spasm by increasing alpha adrenergic activity.

Encyclopedias have been written on the anesthetic management of patients undergoing myocardial revascularization and other adult cardiac surgical procedures. However, some common, but often overlooked, principles remain:

1) Heparin should be given through a central line and its effect documented prior to going on bypass. Cardiopulmonary bypass in the unheparinized patient is a catastrophe.

2) Protamine is both a myocardial depressant and a vasodilator (4). Protamine anaphylaxis needs to be considered especially in patients who are on insulin preparations containing protamine and in patients who have had a vasectomy. Protamine anaphylaxis produces precipitous hypotension and profound hypovolemia. Large doses of epinephrine, e.g. 1-5 mg push, have been reported to be necessary to resuscitate the patient. Immediate reinstitution of cardiopulmonary bypass may be life saving. Giving protamine either directly into the aorta or through an LA line may decrease the incidence but will not totally prevent the occurrence.

3) The multiple array of medications drawn up by the anesthesiologist and the similarity between ampules, e.g. Protamine and Metubine leads to medication errors!

4) Although the V5 lead has become well known to everyone, lead II is better for diagnosing arrhythmias.

5) Atrial manipulation may cause atrial fibrillation when the venous cannula is inserted, especially in the face of hypovolemia. If hemodynamic instability occurs, synchronous cardioversion with 5-10 watt/seconds may be necessary. The quickest and most reliable method available to diagnose atrial fibrillation is direct observation of the atria.

6) When going on bypass, not only must the principles of extracorporeal circulation be remembered but also the awareness that pump mishaps can occur. If something is not right, get off bypass at once (5).

7) Hypovolemia may occur when going on bypass. Hypotension and an empty, beating heart, may precipitate severe myocardial ischemia.

8) When the aortic cross-clamp is placed or when cardioplegia solutions are infused into the aortic root, left ventricular overdistention may occur acutely because of aortic insufficiency or more slowly because of increased myocardial venous return into the left ventricle. This can be recognized by the PA, LA, or CVP abruptly increasing. The surgeon may decompress the heart by squeezing blood

from the heart or by introducing a left ventricular drain (sump). In addition, when going on total bypass, improper placement of the atrial cannula(e), may produce venous obstruction. An abrupt increase in superior vena caval pressure, swelling of the head, or scleral edema may occur.

9) The surgeon may place a partial occluding clamp on the aorta prior to doing the proximal anastomoses. This clamp can partially occlude the orifice to the left coronary artery with sudden ischemic changes or can severely occlude the aorta (recognized by a damped arterial trace).

10) Various forms of myocardial protection are employed (6) during total bypass. Myocardial temperature may be monitored. If it is not, myocardial activity needs to be followed and when any is noted, additional cardioplegia needs to be administered.

11) The minimal acceptable mean arterial pressure during bypass (7) is an ongoing controversy. There is no single answer, nor are there any absolute numbers. However, oxygen requirements of organs vary with temperature. Flow is often more important than pressure. Often, the pump technician will dramatically decrease the flow - 1.4-1.6 L/m^2 and a MAP of 30 occurs. Frequently, by increasing the flow to 2 L/m^2 a MAP of 50 is obtained. However, at times a low C.I. is necessary. If increased venous return obscures the surgical field, a lower C.I. will be requested. If myocardial rewarming occurs very rapidly, the same request will ensue. In these situations, a decision needs to be made. In patients with "normal" circulatory systems, (are CAD patients normal?) a MAP of 30 mmHg is said to be satisfactory. However, in a patient with severe carotid artery disease, this may not be so. In this patient, a MAP of 60-70 mmHg may be necessary. In such a patient, cerebral function should be monitored to ensure adequate cerebral blood flow. In patients with severe carotid artery disease, preoperatively the patient should be evaluated to see if certain positions of the head will induce cerebral ischemia. If such is the case, these positions should be avoided intraoperatively.

12) Certain patients are known to have very low peripheral vascular resistance, and these patients will likely have the same low resistance on bypass. Two groups of patients who frequently exhibit

this are: a) patients with aortic insufficiency; b) patients with congenital heart disease. The use of alpha agonists in the face of reasonable organ perfusion needs to be questioned.

13) Temperature monitoring during heart surgery is done because hypothermia is usually employed during bypass to prevent myocardial rewarming and to minimize flow requirements. Rewarming is done to re-establish homeostasis. The patient is frequently cooled to 20-24° C and rewarmed to 36.8°C. Temperature sites employed are perfusate, nasopharyngeal, tympanic, esophageal, bladder, and rectal in an attempt to identify the core temperature. Postoperatively, many of the side effects of hypothermia are lessened, if shivering is prevented and the patient ventilated until normothermia is achieved.

14) Urine output during bypass is usually maintained above 1 cc/kg/hr. However, there is no correlation between bypass oliguria and post bypass renal failure. Intuitively, if urine output is kept at reasonable levels with minimum effort, this seems desirable. It must be remembered that an occasional patient will put out no urine during non pulsatile flow despite every therapeutic maneuver known. In such a situation if a large dose of furosemide is given, little will occur until partial bypass occurs. Then massive diuresis may occur and the catch up game is on for volume. If massive diuresis occurs in the absence of a diuretic, a high blood sugar may be the causative factor.

15) Air may become lodged in the coronary arteries when coming off bypass. Severe ventricular dysfunction may occur along with markedly elevated ST segments. To rid the coronaries of the air (vapor lock), a potent epinephrine infusion is usually successful. The surgeon may also attempt to "milk the air" thru the vessel.

16) Systemic air embolization must be kept in mind whenever the left side of the heart is opened. Should left ventricular ejection occur while the left side is open, massive air embolus may occur. Air may also be trapped in the root of the aorta or in the pulmonary veins. Therefore, careful aspiration of such air is necessary. Hyperinflation of the lungs is helpful in forcing air from the pulmonary veins.

17) With the use of cardioplegia, hyperkalemic myocardial dysfunction

is not uncommon. If hemodynamic instability is present, hyperkalemia may be treated intravenously with:

a) $CaCl_2$ 200-500 mg

b)   Glucose 25 grams and regular Insulin 20 U.

18) Both atrial and ventricular pacing wires are placed intra-operatively at many institutions. These wires may be very useful in diagnosing postop arrhythmias. Ventricular pacing may be utilized if complete heart block occurs. Likewise, atrial pacing may be employed if atrial bradycardia occurs. Rapid atrial pacing may be therapeutic for certain supraventricular tachycardias. A-V sequential pacing is quite useful should complete heart block occur and atrial contraction is needed for hemodynamic stability. Familiarity with a variety of pacemakers is essential for the anesthesiologist (8).

19) Mitral insufficiency, as manifest by a V wave, should be considered if: a) the PA catheter won't "wedge", b) the LA pressure is excessively high, or c) the LA wave form is exaggerated. Frequently, mitral incompetence occurs because of poor ventricular compliance. By decreasing the afterload with nitroprusside or by increasing the compliance with nitroglycerine, the mitral incompetence frequently disappears. Functional mitral insufficiency is much more common than anatomic in today's practice of cardiac anesthesia.

20) A Starling Curve needs to be plotted, at least mentally, when coming off bypass. A left atrial pressure of greater than 12 mmHg is rarely needed in a patient with reasonable LV function. The need for vasopressors will be greatly decreased if careful attention is given to maximizing cardiac performance. If vasopressors, vasodilators, etc. are ineffective, an intra-aortic balloon pump or a left atrial assist device may be utilized (9).

21) Bleeding remains a problem postoperatively. Guidelines for re-entry are helpful in preventing many of the problems of massive transfusions. Cardiac tamponade must be considered anytime hemodynamic stability can't be quickly corrected. The finding of a low cardiac output along with equalization of the CVP, pulmonary artery diastolic pressure, and a left atrial pressure near 20 mmHg makes the diagnosis of tamponade obvious. However, cardiac

tamponade often presents in a variety of ways, and a high index of suspicion must always be present. Once the diagnosis is established, prompt re-exploration is indicated and the anesthetic technique needs to be resuscitative in nature until decompression is obtained.

The subject of anesthesia requirements for specific valvular surgery will be briefly reviewed.

AORTIC STENOSIS

Patients who develop aortic stenosis frequently have a bicuspid valve. The normal valvular area is 2.0 cm^2/m^2; 0.6 - 0.8 cm^2/m^2 represents moderate stenosis; less than 0.5 cm^2/m^2 represents critical obstruction. If the patient develops severe bradycardia and/or hypotension when the catheter is passed through the valve, the diagnosis of critical stenosis has been made. When anesthetizing patients with aortic stenosis, it is imperative to:

1) Maintain an optimal pulse rate of 70-90.
2) Be aware that asystole can occur reflexly during the sternotomy. Have the atropine immediately available.
3) Severe angina, syncope, and congestive failure are the well known triad of this syndrome. Myocardial ischemia despite the absence of atherosclerotic heart disease is a major problem and often precipitated by tachycardia.
4) Hypotension is poorly tolerated and will rapidly lead to "no" tension.
5) If the patient should arrest, CPR will be very difficult because enough pressure needs to be generated in the left ventricle to overcome the stenosis. For example, if there is a 100 mmHg gradient across the aortic valve, to generate a 100 mmHg systolic aortic pressure, a left ventricular pressure of 200 mmHg will be required.
6) Postoperative hypertension is common since these patients often have "normal" LV function. Once the obstruction is relieved, the aorta will see the pressure generated by the left ventricle. Propranolol is often effective.

MITRAL STENOSIS

Information essential to anesthetizing patients with mitral stenosis is: know that the normal mitral valve area is 4-6 cm^2; clinical symptoms occur at an area less than 2.6 cm^2; and critical mitral stenosis occurs at a valve area less than 1.5 cm^2. Classically, myocardial contractility in these patients is normal. However, many patients show areas of dyskinesia or akinesia because of abnormal chordae tendineae. Considerations in managing this group of patients include:

1) Atrial fibrillation is the rule. The absence of fibrillation makes our job much easier.

2) Rate control is necessary. Tachycardia is poorly tolerated.

3) Sick mitrals are intolerant to sedatives.

4) Because of the low cardiac output, these patients become anesthetized very quickly and are easily "blown away".

5) Don't exacerbate pulmonary hypertension.

6) Avoid cardioversion in patients with long standing fibrillation because of the danger of dislodging emboli, especially systemic.

7) Maintain adequate volume.

8) Wedge pressures (LA) do not reflect left ventricular end diastolic pressures.

9) Postop right heart failure is more common than left heart failure. (CVP may be more important than the wedge pressure.)

10) Low cardiac output syndrome postoperatively often requires aggressive management employing maximum monitoring.

AORTIC INSUFFICIENCY

Aortic insufficiency is usually caused by rheumatic heart disease and endocarditis or by aortic root dissection. In the management of such patients, it is important to:

1) Avoid increases in afterload which will increase regurgitant flow thereby decreasing cardiac output.

2) Maintain an elevated heart rate and avoid bradycardia. A slow rate allows increased LV filling which will also produce increased regurgitant flow.

3) Maintain reasonable volume status because of the need to have a reasonably full heart to compensate for the regurgitant fraction.

4) Low SVR may be helpful and can be achieved with vasodilators. However, coronary perfusion is dependent upon the diastolic pressure, and an abrupt lowering of the diastolic pressure can

induce severe myocardial ischemia leading to ventricular fibrillation.

5) Agents which produce severe myocardial depression will increase ventricular distention. However, increased SVR will also increase the distention.

6) When going on bypass be aware of acute left ventricular distention because of retrograde pump flow through the incompetent valve.

7) On bypass, these patients frequently show a low MAP despite a reasonable pump flow.

8) Post-bypass, especially in patients with long standing aortic insufficiency higher than normal filling pressures may be required because of the long standing ventricular distention.

MITRAL INSUFFICIENCY

Mitral insufficiency may develop because of abnormalities of the:

1) mitral valve leaflets secondary to rheumatic disease.

2) papillary muscle or chordae tendineae secondary to:
   a) mitral valve prolapse
   b) myocardial ischemia or infarction

3) annulus secondary to
   a) left ventricular distention - "functional M.I."
   b) prosthetic perivalvular leak
   c) left atrial distention - adult atrial septal defect.

   It is important to:

1) Keep the peripheral resistance low to decrease the degree of mitral regurgitation.

2) Maintain an elevated heart rate and avoid bradycardia.

3) Remember that if a Swan-Ganz catheter is placed prior to induction, the catheter "will not wedge" because of the "V" waves. However, a Swan-Ganz can be a useful guide in determining the degree of regurgitation by following the size of the V wave.

4) Be prepared to handle a very sick hemodynamically unstable patient if the mitral regurgitation is due to papillary dysfunction secondary to a myocardial infarction. These patients may well require an intra-aortic balloon pump post bypass.

Remember - heart valves may fail postoperatively. Once again a high index of suspicion is necessary if prompt corrective measures are to take place.   Problem encountered for tricuspid valve, pulmonary valve, or multiple valve surgery will not be covered in this lecture.

Any discussion of anesthesia for adult cardiac surgery will be incomplete.   However, I would be remiss if I did not discuss anesthetic problems encountered in patients undergoing "redo" surgery.   The valves fail, or the grafts occlude.   Some common problems are:

1) Line placement may be a problem because of occluded or anatomically distorted vessels.
2) The saw may cut through the right ventricle, adhered to the sternum, during the sternal split.   Severe adhesions are anticipated and femoral cannulation before the sternal split may be advisable. Heparin should be immediately available to crash on bypass through a maze of adhesions.
3) Freeing up the heart is often time consuming and requires various surgical manipulations causing zero cardiac output.   Constant attention and a close relationship between surgeon and anesthesiologist are necessary if the surgeon is to "free up" the heart safely.
4) This is one circumstance where pre-pump blood transfusion may be necessary.

THORACIC ANEURYSM

One of the most challenging cases to confront the anesthesiologist is a thoracic aneurysm.   Preoperatively, it is imperative to know the location and extent of the aneurysm.   The aneurysm may dissect proximally to involve the aortic valve.   The aneurysm discussed will involve only the thoracic aorta just distal to the subclavian artery.   The etiology of such an aneurysm is usually traumatic or arteriosclerotic.   The chest x-ray and angiogram should be reviewed for tracheal compression and/or deviation and to assess any distortion of the major vessels which may make line placement difficult.   The technique to be employed for perfusing the lower body needs to be known in order to make rational decisions about monitoring.

The methods employed include:
1) Cross clamping the aorta - no distal flow.
2) Subclavian artery - femoral artery shunt (Gott shunt).
3) Femoral artery - femoral vein partial bypass.

4) Left atrial to femoral artery bypass.

The left femoral artery is usually chosen by the surgeon for cannulation if a bypass is to be employed. If such is the case, an arterial line should be placed in the right femoral artery to determine lower body perfusion pressure. The right radial artery should also be cannulated to measure upper body perfusion pressure. The left radial is to be avoided because the aneurysm may involve the subclavian artery. The endotracheal tube should preferably be a left sided double-lumen tube. The reasons for the double-lumen tube are:

1) Better surgical exposure.

2) Less postop pulmonary dysfunction because of less hemorrhage and less parenchymal damage to the left lung caused by traction.

3) Protection of the right lung from bleeding from the opposite lung.

Severe hypertension is likely to occur when the surgeon cross clamps the proximal aorta. Deepening the anesthesia and lowering the BP by nitroprusside or other pharmacologic agent may prevent a stroke or acute pulmonary edema. Renal dysfunction because of lack of adequate renal flow may occur. Various regimens are used to prevent postop renal failure but all are at best intuitive in nature.

Postop problems associated with the repair of a thoracic aneurysm include stroke, congestive heart failure, bleeding, hypoxemia. Renal dysfunction is not unexpected because of the nature of the surgery. The extent of the dissection may impair intestinal blood flow and postop intestinal ischemia may occur. A devastating complication is paraplegia. Spinal cord blood flow usually occurs from the vertebral and anterior spinal arteries. However, in a small percentage of patients (approximately 7%) the blood supply comes from one major anterior spinal artery (radicular magna artery) at T7 (10). If the aneurysm involves this artery and the artery is sacrificed, paraplegia may develop. No technique as yet has been successful in preventing this complication (11). The incidence of this complication remains at about 7% regardless of variations in treatment. The left phrenic nerve may be injured during the surgical procedure and cause a paralyzed left diaphragm.

CHRONIC TAMPONADE AND CONSTRICTIVE PERICARDITIS

Chronic tamponade is more commonly seen with today's aggressive care for both malignancies and renal failure. Classical findings for chronic

124

tamponade include elevated central venous pressure, low blood pressure
with decreased pulse pressure, and muffled heart sounds. The principles
of anesthetic management are quite simple.

1) Keep the heart rate fast.

2) Keep the heart full.

3) Keep the patient vasoconstricted.

If these principles are followed and the anesthesiologist stays
alert, success should be assured. However, because of the concomitant
disease, these patients are usually Class IV or V patients.

Constrictive pericarditis is another entity which can be a real
challenge. The surgeon must be meticulous in his dissection to release
the adhesions. Hypotension and arrhythmias are common because of
mechanical obstruction. In addition, bleeding may be a complicating
factor. The heart rate and volume must be maintained. A frightening
unexplained complication may occur when long standing constrictive
pericarditis is relieved. Abrupt cardiac dilatation may occur with
severe decompensation. Underlying cardiomyopathy may be the cause.
However, massive amounts of inotropics, including $CaCl_2$, isuprel, and/or
epinephrine will be required. Despite all out aggressive therapy, a
successful resuscitation may not occur.

REFERENCES

1. Kennedy, J.W., Kaiser, G.C., et al. J. Thorac. Cardiovasc. Surg.
    80:876, 1980.
2. Slogoff, S. and Keats, A.S. Anesthesiology 62:107, 1985.
3. Cheng, T.O. Chest 86:918, 1984.
4. Shapiro, N., Schaff, H.V., et al. J. Thorac. Cardiovasc. Surg.
    84:505, 1982.
5. Stoney, W.S., Alford, W.C., et al. Ann. Thorac. Surg. 29:336,
    1980.
6. Buckberg, G.D. J. Thorac. Cardiovasc. Surg. 77:803, 1979.
7. Govier, A., Reves, J.G., et al. Ann. Thorac. Surg. 38:592, 1984.
8. Ludmer, P.L. and Goldschlager, N. N.E.J.M. 311:1671, 1984.
9. McGee, M.G., Zellgett, S.L., et al. Am. J. Cardiol. 46:135, 1980.
10. DeBakey, M.E., et al. J. Cardiovasc. Surg. 19:57, 1978.
11. Laschinger, J.E., Cunningham, J.N., et al. Ann. Thorac. Surg.
    38:500, 1984.

THE RENIN-ANGIOTENSIN SYSTEM IN ANESTHESIA

E.D. MILLER, JR.

The renin-angiotensin system has received considerable attention in the last several years and is one of a variety of vasoactive substances that are known to be important in controlling blood pressure. The presentation will focus on how the various aspects of the renin-angiotensin system may have important implications for the anesthesiologist. It should be remembered, though, that this is only one of many vasoactive substances and may be a model with which to look at other agents that are known to affect blood pressure. Certainly with the newer information that is now available and the recently synthesized drugs that affect the renin-angiotensin system, we, as anesthesiologists, are now seeing patients who are being treated with these agents both prior to operation and immediately after operation.

First, let us examine the renin-angiotensin system. Renin is an enzyme that is released from the kidney under a variety of stimuli. Once released into the circulation, renin acts on substrate, angiotensinogen formed in the liver, and cleaves off ten amino acids which form the peptide angiotensin I. Angiotensin I has no known physiologic properties and is converted to angiotensin II in a single pass through the lung. The conversion of the ten amino acids, angiotensin I, to eight amino acids, angiotensin II, occurs by cleavage of two amino acids from the angiotensin I by an enzyme called converting enzyme that is located in the endothelium of the pulmonary vasculature. Angiotensin II has a variety of properties that make it important in blood pressure control. These include constriction of arterioles, stimulation of aldosterone secretion, potentiation of thirst, potentiation of catecholamine release, and a variety of other stimulatory properties (1).

The mechanisms that are known to release renin from the afferent arteriole of the kidney include a decrease in the afferent arteriolar pressure (called the baroreceptor theory), changes in sodium which is delivered to the distal nephron (called the macula densa theory), and neurogenic control, that is, stimulation of the nerves that cause the kidney to release renin. As can be seen, these mechanisms are all involved in the regulation of the volume and pressure status of the animal or the human.

Over the past twenty years, a variety of inhibitors of the renin-angiotensin system have been produced. Significant clinical agents that have been used to alter the renin-angiotensin system have focused on either a competitive inhibitor of angiotensin II, such as the peptide saralasin, or agents which inhibit the conversion of angiotensin I to angiotensin II by blocking converting enzyme, such as captopril and the recently released agent, enalpril.

What significance do these various inhibitors have? By use of these inhibitors one can now determine precisely the importance of the renin-angiotensin system in physiologic control, which has not been possible in the past (2). For example, the measurement of plasma renin activity in an in vitro test could only determine that renin was present. However, the importance of that renin could not be quantitated. For example, the use of the inhibitors of the renin-angiotensin system was applied in renovascular hypertension. It was demonstrated that the relationship between the increase in blood pressure and the rise in the plasma renin activity were not two independent variables. Rather, the rise in blood pressure was due to the increase in renin, and this was demonstrated by using a converting enzyme inhibitor (3). Using a similar technique, animals made severely sodium depleted and therefore had high plasma renin activity had a significant degree of blood pressure support due to activation of the renin-angiotensin system. It was demonstrated further that angiotensin II was a specific feedback on the release of renin from the kidney (4).

What is the clinical significance of these findings? Various studies demonstrated that during anesthesia, plasma renin activity did not increase; however, when one used an inhibitor of the renin-angiotensin system, both in normal sodium and in salt-depleted animals, there was a significant decrease in blood pressure (5). This finding, in the face of a normal plasma renin activity, again demonstrated the importance of using inhibitors of the renin-angiotensin system to determine the importance of the role of that system.

How do anesthetic agents affect the renin-angiotensin system? It was possible that anesthetic agents altered converting enzyme activity. Both in vitro and in vivo studies have now conclusively shown that the commonly used inhalation agents do not alter converting enzyme activity (6). Furthermore, activation of the renin-angiotensin system is still possible during anesthesia. Several studies have now demonstrated the fact that with controlled hypotension there is significant elevation in plasma renin activity and that this activity is important in blood pressure control (7). Not only is blood pressure control an important factor, but probably more important is the distribution of that blood flow within the animal (8). Other examples of where the renin-angiotensin system has a significant role would be during times of acute hemorrhage where the renin-angiotensin system is maximally stimulated in an attempt to restore volume. At least with two anesthetic agents there does not appear to be a significant difference in this activation (9).

What is the clinical significance of the recently synthesized inhibitors of the renin-angiotensin system? Their clinical roles have now been demonstrated in a few very specific areas. These include deliberate hypotension, postoperative hypertension, and blood flow to various organs. A detailed examination of each one of these is indicated.

Deliberate hypotension is known to stimulate the renin-angiotensin system significantly. Early studies show that not only was there a increase in plasma renin activity when sodium nitroprusside was used to induce hypotension, but there was also a rebound hypertension that occurred with a discontinuation of sodium nitroprusside (10). This rebound hypertension was due to circulating levels of angiotensin II. Subsequent studies have shown that with blockade of the renin-angiotensin system there is no significant rebound hypertension (11). It has also been demonstrated that propranolol can significantly decrease renin release from the kidney. Both by pretreatment and by intravenous treatment during controlled hypotension plasma renin activity is markedly lowered, and there is a tendency for less sodium nitroprusside to be used to provide the same degree of hypotension (12). More recent studies have shown that with the pretreatment of patients with 3 mg/kg of captopril, the dose of sodium nitroprusside can be markedly decreased and the same degree of hypotension achieved with ease (13).

One of the major problems of treatment of patients in the surgical setting with agents such as captopril is that it is limited because there is no intravenous form of this medication. Recently, enalpril has been released in the oral form, and the intravenous form is available for experimental use. It has been shown that patients, after undergoing coronary surgery, who then develop significant hypertension, can have their hypertension markedly diminished by the intravenous use of enalpril. Not only does blood pressure decrease significantly, but there is a decrease in plasma catacholamines. This decrease in plasma catecholamines is thought to be due to the blockade of the facilitation of release of catecholamines by angiotensin II. With the decreased amounts of angiotensin II secondary to the enalpril treatment, blood pressure is diminished by this mechanism as well (14).

A third area where treatment with a converting enzyme inhibitor has proven effective is in the cross-clamping of the thoracic aorta. With surgical operations on the thoracic aorta, blood supply to the various organs may be markedly diminished during the time of cross-clamp. One of the major concerns is blood flow to the kidneys, the liver, and the spinal cord. Initial studies suggest that blood flow can be markedly improved to these regions after the cross-clamp on the thoracic aorta is removed. This would suggest that locally active angiotensin II produces an intense vasoconstriction that persists after the release of the cross-clamp. Pretreatment with converting enzyme inhibitors seems to improve blood flow to these organs. Studies are in progress to determine whether this improved flow will result in improved function (15).

Inhibitors of the renin-angiotensin system will continue to be synthesized. Their role in various physiologic and pathologic states remains to be determined. It is well-established now that only through the use of inhibitors of the system can one really determine the importance of the renin-angiotensin system in controlling blood pressure, blood flow, and organ function.

REFERENCES

1. Haber, E., Sancho, J., Re, R., and Barger, A.C. Clin Sci Mol Med 48:495-502, 1975.

2. Bumpus, F.M., Sen, S., Smeby, R., Sweet, C.S., Ferrario, C.M., and Khosla, M.C. Circ Res 32 (Suppl 1):150-160, 1973.

3. Miller, E.D., Samuels, A., Haber, E., and Barger, A.C. Science 117:1108-1109, 1972.

4. Samuels, A., Miller, E.D., Fray, J., Haber, E., and Barger, A.C. Fed Proc 35:2512-2520, 1976.

5. Miller, E.D., Longnecker, D.E., and Peach, M.J. Anesthesiology 48:399-403, 1978.

6. Miller, E.D., Gianfagna, W., Ackerly, J.A., and Peach, M.J. Anesthesiology 50:88-92, 1979.

7. Miller, E.D., Ackerly, J.A., Vaughan, E.D., Peach, M.J., and Epstein, R.M. Anesthesiology 47:257-263, 1977.

8. Miller, E.D., Delaney, T.J., and Beckman, J.J. Anesthesiology 54:199-203, 1981.

9. Miller, E.D., Longnecker, D.E., and Peach, M.J. Circ Shock 6:271-276, 1979.

10. Khambatta, H.J., Stone, J.G., and Khan, E. Anesthesiology 51:127-130, 1979.

11. Delaney, T.J. and Miller E.D. Anesthesiology 52:154-156, 1980.

12. Marshall, W.K., Bedford, R.F., Arnold, W.P., and Miller, E.D. Anesthesiology 55:277-280, 1981.

13. Woodside, J.R., Garner, L., Bedford, R.F., Sussman, M.D., Miller, E.D., Longnecker, D.E., and Epstein, R.M. Anesthesiology 60:413-417, 1984.

14. Joob, A.W., Harmen, P.K., Miller, E.D., Ayers, C.R., and Mentzer, R.M. Society of Cardiovascular Anesthesiologists, May, 1986, Montreal, Canada.

15. Joob, A.W., Harmen, P.K., Freelender, A.E., Miller, E.D., and Kron, I.L. Surg Forum 35:318-319, 1984.

MECHANISMS OF MYOCARDIAL ISCHEMIA DURING ANESTHESIA.

Sebastian Reiz MD, PhD.

Careful monitoring and control of systemic blood pressure and heart rate still seem to be the most effective means of avoiding perioperative myocardial ischemia. In a comparison of the predicitive value for ischemia of the commonly measured hemodynamic variables, Lieberman and co-workers (1) found the systolic blood pressure to have the highest predicitive value of positive tests (79%) and the highest efficiency (84%). In comparison, an elevated pulmonary capillary wedge pressure had an efficiency to predict ischemia of 55% only. These authors found the combination of decreased systolic blood pressure (more than 30% below the awake value or less than 90 mm Hg) and tachycardia to be the variables most commonly associated with ischemia. These findings are partly in contrast with those obtained by Slogoff and Keats (2). They found that perioperative ischemia correlated with tachycardia and hypertension rather than hypotension. More intriguing in this study was that more than half the ischemic episodes were temporally unassociated with hemodynamic abnormalities. This suggests that other mechanisms for ischemia than those generally recognized, may be active during anesthesia and surgery.

Until recently, it has been believed that an increase in oxygen demand in an area supplied via a flow limiting coronary artery stenosis was usually responsible for myocardial ischemia. Studies are now appearing, in which it is demonstrated that the effects of distensibility upon stenosis resistance, coronary vasospasm and redistribution of regional myocardial blood flow might be important mechanisms for perioperative myocardial ischemia. The role of coronary vasodilating anesthetic agents (i.e. isoflurane) in myocardial ischemia is covered in detail in another paper in this publication. This presentation will therefore concentrate on the importance of the two former mechanisms, in particular coronary vasospasm.

Stenosis resistance is constant in rigid stenoses but varies in stenoses incorporating an elastic element. When distal pressure increases with a rigid stenosis, the pressure gradient across the stenosis is reduced and flow decreases. Conversely, when distal pressure decreases, flow across the stenosis increases. With a distensible stenosis, increase in distal pressure may cause an increase in stenosis area. Consequently, flow may increase despite a decreased pressure gradient. Conversely, if distal pressure falls, flow may decrease. This mechanism is effective in extremely tight stenoses incorporating an elastic element of the vascular wall and is one factor that may explain the poor efficiency of increased pulmonary capillary wedge pressure in the Lieberman study (1).

Slogoff and Keats (2) described new ST-segment changes typical of ischemia in almost 20% of their patients upon arrival in the operating room. The patients were often free from angina and their hemodynamic variables were within normal limits. It has been suggested, that these patients may have had coronary vasospasm (3). Maseri's group has established the importance of coronary vasospasm in stable angina pectoris (4). Continuous monitoring of the ECG in such patients has documented that ST-segment depression (unlike elevation seen in coronary vasospasm and angina of the Variant type) preceeds changes in heart rate and blood pressure and is associated with hypoperfusion on scintigraphy. One anatomical basis for coronary vasospasm is an eccentric coronary artery stenosis, leaving a portion of the vessel wall which remains reactive. Furthermore, recent reports describe hyperreactivity in elastic stenoses, particularly following noradrenergic stimulation (5).

Our group compared patients with coronary artery disease who became ischemic during laryngoscopy and intubation with those who did not. Patients were premedicated with morphine and induced with fentanyl, thiopentone and enflurane or isoflurane in nitrous oxide/oxygen to a mean arterial pressure approximately 70% of their awake value. Systemic, pulmonary and coronary hemodynamics were followed from before laryngoscopy until 10 min post intubation. Blood samples for myocardial lactate balance studies, 12-lead ECG-s and cardiokymograms were obtained at regular intervals. Patients who became ischemic (n=30) demonstrated immediate reductions in coronary blood flow following upon laryngoscopy (i.e. within a few heart beats). In contrast, non-ischemic patients (n=20) had no such change. Strikingly, the reduction in coronary blood flow preceeded any increase in systemic blood pressure, heart rate or pulmonary artery diastolic pressure (Fig 1). When the laryngoscope was removed, coronary blood flow returned to control levels in the ischemic patients. The systemic and pulmonary hemodynamic effects of laryngoscopy and intubation were similar in ischemic and non-ischemic patients (Fig 2). Furthermore, the 12-lead ECG was abnormal in one third of the ischemic patients only.

Fig 1. With laryngoscopy, coronary sinus blood flow (CSF) decreased by about 40% prior to any change in arterial pressure, heart rate or pulmonary artery diastolic pressure. With termination of the intubation, blood flow returned to control levels. An upward shift of the mixed blood-indicator resistance curve denotes flow reduction. Neurogenically mediated vasospasm is the most likely cause for the decrease in coronary blood flow.

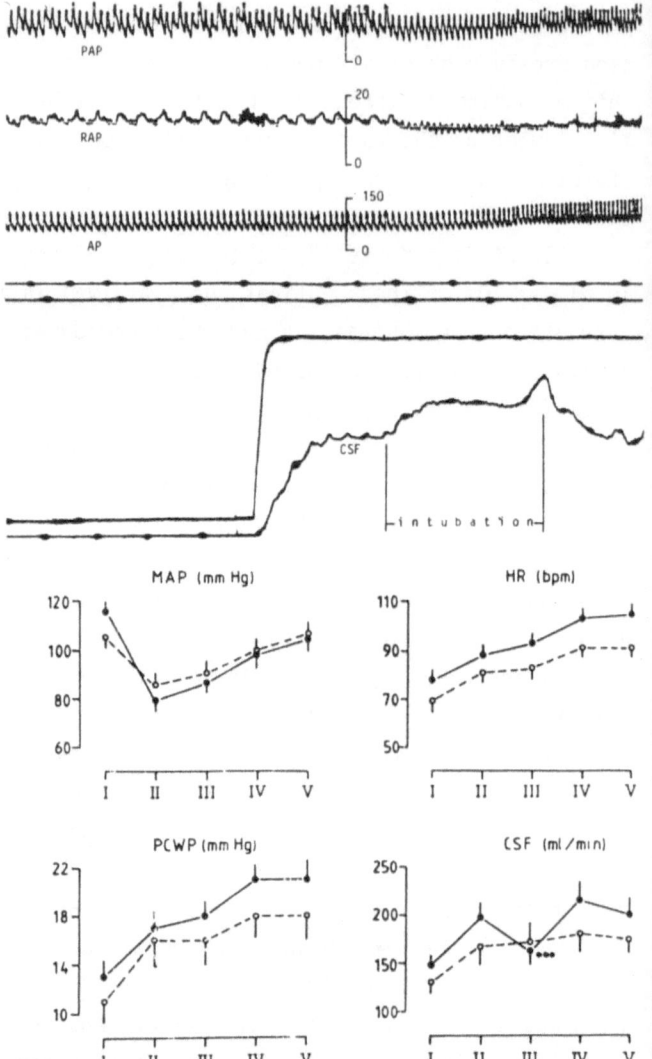

Fig 2. Effects of laryngoscopy and intubation on systemic hemodynamics and coronary sinus blood flow in patients with coronary artery disease. Solid lines denote patients who became ischemic (n=30), broken lines non-ischemic patients (n=20). I - awake, II - immediately before laryngoscopy, III - during laryngoscopy, IV - at the end of intubation, V - at the time of maximal hemodynamic changes.
*** $p < 0.001$ compared with non-ischemic patients from II to III.

It is probable that neurogenically mediated vasoconstriction is responsible for the rapid initial decline in coronary blood flow. One would have expected an increase in blood flow in conjunction with the increase in myocardial oxygen demand during the subsequent period. Technically, it was not possible to obtain blood gases during the study period. However, Moffitt and colleagues observed an increase in myocardial oxygen extraction without change in coronary blood flow during laryngoscopy and intubation of patients scheduled to undergo coronary artery bypass grafting (6). They did not report any patient to be ischemic in this study. It is possible that all of these data are consistent with increased coronary vascular tone. Thus, decreased supply of oxygen, rather than increased demand seems to be the dominating mechanism for ischemia during laryngoscopy and intubation.

Our study was continued during the time of surgery. Like in previous studies, myocardial ischemia recorded during surgery, was most commonly associated with the combination of hypertension, tachycardia and increased pulmonary capillary wedge pressure, hence a combination of increased demand and impaired supply of oxygen to the myocardium. Wilkinson and co-workers studied the effects of anesthesia and surgery during halothane or high dose morphine anesthesia on coronary hemodynamics and myocardial oxygenation of patients undergoing coronary bypass grafting (7). The authors found that sternotomy during morphine anesthesia was associated with significantly greater increase in blood pressure than during halothane anesthesia. There was a comparable increase in coronary blood flow, but myocardial oxygen extraction increased more in the halothane group. This implies an inability in the patients anesthetized with halothane to increase coronary blood flow in proportion to demand. Ischemia developed in 9 of 14 halothane patients and in 4 of 12 administered morphine. In similar patients studied by Hilfiker and colleagues, sternotomy during halothane anesthesia was not associated with ischemia in any patient (8). Some of the patients in our study developed ischemia without changes in the peripheral determinants of the myocardial supply/demand ratio for oxygen and despite the use of an anesthetic agent which produces cardiodepression. Typically, these patients demonstrated pronounced reductions in coronary blood flow parallelling the ECG changes (Fig 3). These results support the assumption of coronary vasospasm as an active mechanism for ischemia during surgery.

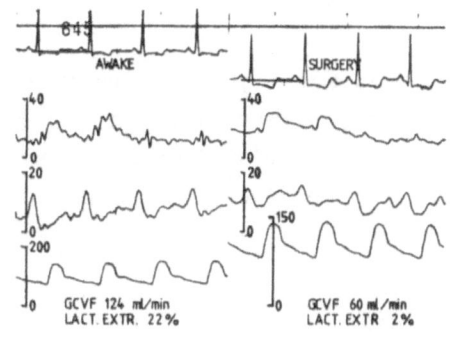

Fig 3. V5 ECG, pulmonary arterial, right atrial and systemic arterial pressure (top to bottom) in one patient before (left) and during abdominal surgery (right) under isoflurane-fentanyl-nitrous oxide/oxygen anesthesia. Despite comparable blood pressure, heart rate and filling pressure, great cardiac venous blood flow (GCVF) had decreased to half, myocardial lactate extraction fallen from 22 to 2% and ischemic ECG changes appeared. The findings suggest coronary vasospasm.

Larsen and coworkers performed random studies on the effects of enflurane versus isoflurane/nitrous oxide-oxygen anesthesia on coronary hemodynamics and
myocardial oxygenation of patients subjected to coronary artery bypass grafting (9). The effects of the anesthetic agents were similar. Coronary blood
flow decreased with perfusion pressure, although isoflurane produced a lesser
reduction than enflurane (Fig 4). As expected from the previously documented
coronary vasodilating properties of the agents (10, 11), a pronounced and comparable increase in coronary sinus oxygen content was observed. With sternotomy, important differences became obvious. Sungery during enflurane anesthesia
was associated with a return of myocardial blood flow and coronary sinus oxygen
content, hence a normal autoregulatory response to increased demand for oxygen.
No ischemia was observed. With isoflurane, coronary venous oxygen content remained elevated, suggesting persisting coronary vasodilation and intereference
with the normal autoregulatory response to the increase in myocardial oxygen
demand (Fig 4). Three of ten isoflurane patients became ischemic.

Fig 4. Effects of anesthesia and sternotomy on hemodynamics and myocardial
nutrition during enflurane-nitrous
oxide or isoflurane-nitrous oxide
anesthesia in patients with coronary
artery disease. Heart rate and blood
pressure response were similar in the
two groups of patients. Coronary sinus
oxygen content remained elevated with
sternotomy during isoflurane anesthesia
despite decreasing lactate extraction.
Plotted from data by Larsen et al (9)

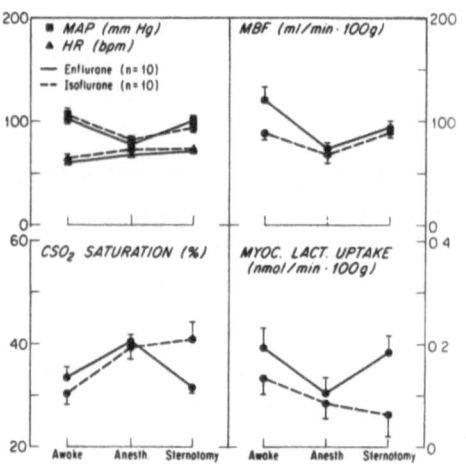

In summary, the pertubations of laryngoscopy and intubation and major surgery may produce changes in coronary vascular tone and myocardial oxygenation
which are unrelated to the changes in systemic hemodynamics or filling pressure
It seems as if hyperperfusion and hypoperfusion of areas of the myocardium may
coexist.

REFERENCES

1. Lieberman, R.W., Orkin, F.K., Jobes, D.R. and Schwartz, A.J.:Anesthesiology. 59: 36-41, 1983.
2. Slogoff, S. and Keats, A.S.: Anesthesiology 62: 107-114, 1985.
3. Lowenstein, E.: Anesthesiology 62: 103-106, 1985 (editorial).
4. Deanfield, J.E., Maseri, A., Selwyn, A.P., et al: Lancet 2: 753-758, 1983.
5. Mudge, G.H.Jr., Grossman, W., Mills, R.M. Jr., et al: N. Engl. J. Med. 295: 1333-1337, 1976.
6. Moffitt, E.A., Sethna, D.H., Bussell, J.A., et al: Can. Anaesth. Soc. J. 32: 105-111, 1985.
7. Wilkinson, P.L., Hamilton, W.K., Moyers, J.R., et al: J. Thorac. Cardiovasc. Surg. 82: 372-380, 1981.
8. Hilfiker, O., Larsen, R., Sonntag, H. Br. J. Anaesthesia 55: 927-932, 1983.
9. Larsen, R., Hilfiker, O., Merkel, G., et al. Anesthesiology 61: A4, 1984.
10. Rydvall, A., Häggmark, S., Nyhman, H., et al. Acta Anaesthesiol. Scand. 28: 690-695, 1984.
11. Reiz, S., Bålfors, E., Sørensen,M.B., et al. Anesthesiology 59: 91-97, 1983.

MECHANISMS AND MANAGEMENT OF CARDIAC ARRHYTHMIAS

RONALD L. KATZ

FREQUENCY OF ARRHYTHMIAS

This paper will deal with cardiac arrhythmias in the perioperative period, except for those associated with cardiac surgery. Although there were case reports concerning cardiac arrhythmias in the operating room as early as the 1900s (Levy and Lewis 1911-12), it was not until the past 10-20 years that large series of patients were studied to determine the incidence of arrhythmias. In 1962, Dodd and associates reported a 30% incidence of cardiac arrhythmias in 569 patients. It should be pointed out that in this study an oscilloscope was used and that permanent tracings were not made. Thus, it may be that a significant number of arrhythmias were missed. On the other hand, one can argue that if the duration of arrhythmia was so brief so as not to be noted, then the clinical significance is minimal. The arrhythmias which were observed were slow, super-ventricular rhythms (atrial rhythms, AV junctional rhythm, wandering pacemaker, sinus arrest with supra-ventricular escape beats). These occurred in 16% of the patients. Premature ventricular contractions were observed in 12.5% of the patients. The incidence of arrhythmias was higher in patients with heart disease than in those without, being 51% in the former and 20% in the latter. It is of interest that contrary to the clinical impressions of many people, there were no significant differences in the frequency fo arrhythmias with ether, nitrous oxide, halothane, cyclopropane, or spinal (tetracaine).

In 1966, Reinikainen and Pontinen determined the frequency of arrhythmias in approximately 1,200 patients. They noted that with halothane, 13% of the patients developed arrhythmias during maintenance. With epidural anesthesia, with prilocaine, the incidence was 18%, whereas with neuroleptanalgesia, the incidence was 16%. In addition to these arrhythmias seen during maintenance, arrhythmias were also seen associated with endotracheal intubation and varied from 25-61%, depending upon the circumstances associated with the intubation.

A year later, in 1967, Kuner et al. reported results in patients in whom a Holter monitor was used to continuously record the electrocardiogram on magnetic tape. The tape was then analyzed after the operation. These workers studied 154 patients. Arrhythmias were noted during operation in 62% of the patients. In this study, 8% of the patients had arrhythmias prior to induction of anesthesia. The most common arrhythmias seen were slow, supraventricular rhythms as defined above, with premature ventricular contractions next most common. In this study, there were no differences between the frequency of new arrhythmias in patients with and patients without preoperative arrhythmias. There were no significant differences between the incidence of arrhythmias in patients with and patients without pre-existing heart disease. This finding is in contrast to most other studies of perioperative arrhythmias. It may be that the arrhythmic frequency was so high in this study that significant differences were not observed. As has been observed by others, arrhythmias in this study were as frequent during general anesthesia as during regional anesthesia. Arrhythmias were more frequent in patients undergoing operations which lasted more than 3 hours than in patients undergoing shorter operations. It may be that the greater duration of operation was associated with a more serious type of operation and a patient who was in poorer status than the patients undergoing brief operations. However, the authors stated that they could find no correlation between physical status and frequency of arrhythmias. This study is, in general, a puzzling one, since it differs from many of the other studies performed.

In perhaps the largest study of perioperative arrhythmias carried out, Vanick and Davis in 1968 published their study of more than 5,000 patients. They found that the frequency of arrhythmias was highest (34%) in patients with known preoperative heart disease, but without preoperative arrhythmias, was next highest (27%) in patients with known preoperative arrhythmias (these intraoperative arrhythmias being different from the ones the patients had preoperatively) and the lowest incidence of arrhythmias (16.3%) occurred in patients with no known preoperative heart disease. As in previous studies, the most common arrhythmias were slow, supra-ventricular rhythms, with premature ventricular contractions the next most common. These workers noted that arrhythmias were less common in patients under 30 years of age, and that 20% of all arrhythmias occurred within the first 5 minutes of anesthesia (i.e., during induction). There was no difference in the frequency of arrhythmias during halothane anesthesia (17%) compared with regional anesthesia (19%). The incidence of arrhythmias with cyclopropane was higher (25%); however, these authors pointed out that their experience with cyclopropane was limited, and it may well be that this accounted for the somewhat higher incidence with cyclopropane. Certainly, this figure of 25% is significantly higher than in the author's own studies with cyclopropane, with which they were quite familiar. Vanick and Davis also noted differences in frequency of arrhythmias in patients on digitalis. The incidence in these patients was 43%, as compared to 17% in patients not receiving digitalis. This raises the question of whether the digitalis per se is responsible for the arrhythmias, or the patient's condition responsible for his being on the digitalis accounted for the arrhythmias. Although it is not possible to be absolutely certain, it appears likely that both were contributing factors. We have observed a higher incidence of arrhythmias in healthy patients placed on digitalis prophylactically than in a similar group of patients not receiving digitalis. However, the differences between these two groups are not great enough to explain the large differences in frequency found by Vanick and Davis. It is therefore likely that the patient's disease responsible for his being on the digitalis is the most important factor.

In reviewing these studies, certain conclusions may be drawn. One is that the reported incidence of arrhythmias is higher when the ECG is recorded continuously than when it is observed on the oscilloscope. A greater frequency of arrhythmias occurs, (1) in patients who have pre-existing arrhythmias or heart disease, (2) in patients receiving digitalis, and (3) when the operation lasted more than 3 hours. Another important point is the adequacy of respiration. Reinikainen and Pontinen (1966) observed that there were twice as many arrhythmias with spontaneous breathing as with controlled respiration. Although the arterial Pco_2 was not measured, it is tempting to speculate that the CO_2 levels were higher in the spontaneously breathing patients than in those with controlled respiration. Several factors may be involved here: one is that with spontaneous respiration, an elevated carbon dioxide greater than normal may occur and this may cause arrhythmias (see below). Another

factor is that hyperventilation and the associated alkalosis and low
Pco_2 may decrease the frequency of arrhythmias. An additional factor is
that hyperventilation may initiate reflex responses which inhibit cardiac
arrhythmias (Katz and Bigger 1970).

Although it is widely believed that the incidence of arrhythmias
with regional anesthesia is less than with general anesthesia, the
published studies do not support this view. In addition to the studies
mentioned above, Hughes et al. (1966) in dental anesthesia patients
found a substantial incidence of arrhythmias in patients who received
the local anesthetic lidocaine for dental anesthesia. They also observed
that the patient's condition was an important factor. In patients with a
normal cardiovascular system, arrhythmias frequency was 17%, while in
patients with known heart disease, it was 33%.

ANESTHETIC AGENT

Arrhythmias may be due to the anesthetic agent itself (Katz and
Bigger 1970). Indeed, halopropane and teflurane can produce cardiac
arrhythmias in concentrations needed for clinical anesthesia (Stephen
and North 1964, Katz 1965, Artusio et al. 1967). Because of this fact,
neither of these agents is available today. There are other agents, such
as cyclopropane and trichlorethylene (Lurie et al. 1958, Waters et al.
1943) which produce arrhythmias, but usually only when given in concentrations greater than needed for surgical anesthesia. With these agents,
it is usually possible to decrease the concentration to a point at which
the patient is still adequately anesthetized, but without arrhythmias.
Of the more commonly used agents such as halothane, enflurane and nitrous
oxide, arrhythmias are much less common, even in the presence of excessive
depth of anesthesia. In studies of the mechanisms of arrhythmias with
halopropane and cyclopropane, it was clear that there was an important
central nervous system component to the arrhythmia (Katz 1966); a finding
similar to that of Beattie et al. (1928) with chloroform.

ANESTHETIC AGENT AND CARBON DIOXIDE

Perhaps the most common cause of arrhythmias in the past was the
combination of the anesthetic agent and carbon dioxide. There have been
a number of studies in which the level of arterial Pco_2 needed to
produce arrhythmias has been determined. With cyclopropane, the threshold

arterial Pco_2 required was 58 torr with a range of 44 to 72 torr (Price et al. 1958). In another study by the same group (Lurie et al. 1958), the threshold arterial Pco_2 for arrhythmias was 74 torr with a range of 44 to 107 torr. It is known that the threshold Pco_2 needed to produce arrhythmias is inversely related to the concentration of cyclopropane.

In studies with halothane, the threshold arterial Pco_2 required to produce arrhythmias was 92 torr with a range of 60-140 torr (Black et al. 1959). In a recent study by Eicard and Skovsted (1976), the carbon dioxide arrhythmias threshold for halothane was compared with that of fluroxene. These workers observed a mean threshold with halothane of 97 torr with a range of 82-109 torr. These figures are similar to those of Black et al., in which a mean arrhythmias threshold of 92 torr was noted. It was not possible with fluroxene to find an arrhythmia threshold. The mean Pco_2 achieved in fluroxene groups was 108 with a range of 92-115. It is also not possible to demonstrate an arrhythmia threshold Pco_2 level for enflurane.

In animal studies of the mechanism of anesthetic agent-carbon dioxide arrhythmias, it was clearly demonstrated that the sympathetic nervous system played a major role in the genesis of arrhythmias. It is well established than an elevated arterial Pco_2 can increase plasma catecholamine levels. Furthermore, beta adrenergic blockade abolishes these arrhythmias. In addition, treatment such as reserpine, bilateral adrenalectomy or a variety of measures which decrease sympathetic outflow and release of catecholamines prevented the arrhythmias (Katz 1966, Katz and Bigger 1970).

Hypoxia can lead to the release of catecholamines and cardiac arrhythmias. The interaction of anesthetic agent and hypoxia in the production of cardiac arrhythmias has been little studied.

ANESTHETIC AGENT AND CATECHOLAMINES

Although at one time, the most common cause of arrhythmias was a comgination of an anesthetic agent and respiratory acidosis, the situation has probably changed in the past 10 years. The marked emphasis on maintaining adequate ventilation has markedly diminished the frequency of respiratory acidosis during anesthesia. The wide availability of arterial blood gases during operations has made it possible to assure that respiratory acidosis does not occur. Although there have been

great gains in diminishing the frequency of anesthetic agent-carbon
dioxide arrhythmias, the situation is less promising for arrhythmias due
to the interaction of an anesthetic agent and catecholamines. This
interaction of anesthetic agents and adrenergic drugs to produce cardiac
arrhythmias was reviewed 10 years ago (Katz and Epstein 1968). This paper
will summarize the information contained in that review as well as
discuss some of the newer data available. It is well established that if
sufficiently large doses of catecholamines such as epinephrine,
norepinephrine and isoproterenol are injected in unanesthetized patients
or animals, cardiac arrhythmias will occur. It is also well-known that
in the presence of halogenated hydrocarbons or cyclopropane, the dose of
catecholamines required to produce an arrhythmia is markedly diminshed.
The decrease in dose may be to as little as one-tenth of the control dose
required to produce arrhythmias. This phenomenon is referred to as
myocardial sensitization. It is not uncommon to inject catecholamines or
adrenergic drugs intravenously during operations for their vasopressor
effect, for their bronchodilator effect, or to inject these agents locally
to produce vasoconstriction. The anesthetic agents which decrease the
arrhythmia dose of catecholamines (produce sensitization) include
trichloroethylene, ethyl chloride, cyclopropane, halothane, chloroform,
methoxyflurane and fluroxene. These agents are listed in order of
decreasing sensitization in dogs. It is known, however, that there are
differences between dog and man. For example, trichloroethylene is a
more potent sensitizer than cyclopropane in the dog, but in man the
reverse is true.

In addition to epinephrine, norepinephrine, isoproterenol, other
adrenergic drugs capable of producing arrhythmias in the presence of
halogenated hydrocarbons include metaraminol and dopamine. It has been
reported that dopamine is less likely to produce cardiac arrhythmias in
halothane-anesthetized cats than is epinephrine (Katz et al. 1967).
However, in the goat, Zahed and associates (1977) found that dopamine had
no advantages over epinephrine in reversing halothane-induced myocardial
depression in terms of lack of arrhythmias. Our own studies suggest that
man behaves more like the cat than the goat, and that dopamine does have
advantages over epinephrine as well as isoproterenol in terms of its
ability to produce myocardial stimulation, but without causing arrhythmias.
A recently developed adrenergic agent which appears to be fairly specific

in terms of increasing myocardial contractility, but with little effect on heart rate or the production of cardiac arrhythmias is dobutamine. Further studies are necessary to indicate whether dobutamine will live up to its early promise of being capable of stimulating the myocardium without producing arrhythmias.

Ethrane is a newer commonly-used anesthetic which appears to be as safe as, if not safer than, halothane in terms of the development of arrhythmias when epinephrine is injected. Vidouse (1975) continuously infused epinephrine during halothane and enflurane anesthesia. The total amount of epinephrine infused to produce arrhythmias was 123 mg with halothane and 174 mg with enflurane. These differences were not statistically significant; however, since there were only 6 patients in each group, it may well be that with larger groups of patients studied there will be a statistically significant difference. Lippman and Reisner (1974) studied the interaction of enflurane and epinephrine and concluded that epinephrine could safely be used with enflurane. A similar study with similar results was also carried out by Konchigeri et al. (1974).

A greater safety margin with enflurane as compared with halothane was observed in the study of Suzuki et al. (1976). They studied 32 children who received epinephrine while undergoing cleft palate surgery, half of whom received halothane. Fewer arrhythmias were observed with enflurane than with halothane. Although the number of patients studied is rather small, other observations would support the concept that the likelihood of arrhythmias following injection of epinephrine is less than enflurane than it is with halothane. Perhaps the best documented study in this regard is that of Johnston et al. (1976). They studied the effects of epinephrine injected into the oral and nasal submucosa in patients undergoing transnasal hypothesectomy. Their end-point was the dose of epinephrine which produced three or more premature ventricular contractions. These workers calculated the ED_{50} for halothane, enflurane and isoflurane. The ED_{50} of epinephrine during halothane was 2.1 ug/kg, for isoflurane it was 6.7 ug/kg and for enflurane it was 10.9 ug/kg. These workers also noted in halothane anesthetized patients that if epinephrine was injected with lidocaine rather than with saline, the ED_{50} for lidocaine with epinephrine was 3.7 ug/kg as compared to 2.1 ug/kg for epinephrine with saline. They then stated that if one assumed the dose equivalent to one-half the ED_{50} did not produce arrhythmias, then the following amounts of epinephrine could safely be given with various anesthetics. For halothane, they felt that 1 ug/kg of epinephrine in saline was safe, while with isoflurane 3.4 ug/kg of epinephrine in saline was safe. They also suggested that if 0.5% lidocaine was used rather than saline, the maximum safe level could be increased 50%. In our own studies in which lidocaine and epinephrine in various concentrations were intravenously infused during halothane anesthesia, we observed that the protection against arrhythmias with 2% lidocaine was greater than with 0.5% lidocaine. Thus, it may be that when 1 or 2% lidocaine with epinephrine is used, even larger amounts of epinephrine can safely be given. The argument may be somewhat academic in that with both halothane and enflurane, the amounts of epinephrine normally necessary to produce adequate vasoconstriction is usually less than the amount which will produce arrhythmias. Thus, one can conclude that the injection of epinephrine during halothane or enflurane is safe as long as reasonable amounts of epinephrine are used. However, there is no doubt that the use of lidocaine rather than saline and the use of enflurane will provide a greater safety margin or will permit the use of larger doses of epinephrine. It is important to point out that in the work of Johnston et al., the epinephrine was injected into the highly vascular oral and nasal submucosa. Thus, the doses these authors concluded to be safe may be smaller than will be safe when injections are made into less vascular areas (i.e., larger doses of epinephrine can safely be injected into less vascular areas). On the other hand, these doses will not be as safe when injected into more vascular areas, or particularly when given intravenously.

Our own studies of the interaction of catecholamines with halothane, enflurane and isoflurane (Conner, Miller, Katz 1976), support the lesser likelihood of producing arrhythmias with enflurane or isoflurane. In a patient undergoing anesthesia for removal of a pheochromocytoma with enflurane, it was noted that on manipulation of the adrenal tumor to a degree that the systolic arterial blood pressure reached 250 torr, there were no cardiac arrhythmias observed. This can be compared with our previous demonstration that the arrhythmia threshold for halothane varies 175 to 225 torr systolic pressure (Katz and Wolf 1971). In this patient, in whom a systolic pressure of 250 did not produce arrhythmias during enflurane, it was subsequently necessary to turn off the ethrane because of bronchospasm. Upon switching to halothane and with the continued manipulation of the tumor, it was noted that arrhythmias occurred at a systolic arterial pressure of 190 torr, suggesting a lower arrhythmias threshold with halothane than with enflurane. Subsequently, the halothane was discontinued and ethrane was given. Once again, it was possible for the systolic pressure to reach 260 torr without the development of arrhythmias. In a similar kind of situation, the authors are also aware of a patient who underwent pheochromocytoma removal under enflurane anesthesia. In this patient, the systolic arterial pressure reached 350 torr, but cardiac arrhythmias were not observed.

In studies in children it has been reported that epinephrine can safely be used with halothane in the following doses: (1) in infants 3.5 ug/kg, (2) in children up to the age of two years, 2.5 ug/kg, and (3) in childrn greater than two years, 1.45 ug/kg (Melgrave 1970).

Ideally, the use of epinephrine should be avoided. However, if it must be injected subcutaneously for local hemostasis, arrhythmias can be prevented if certain precautions are taken. An epinephrine concentration of 1:100,000 or 1:200,000 should be used. In most cases, it is possible to achieve adequate hemostasis with the leser concentration. In the adult, a total dose not greater than 10 ml of 1:100,000 every 10 min., nor more than 30 ml/hr are safe with halothane, trichlorethylene and methoxyflurane. If a 1:200,000 concentration is used, then twice the amount of epinephrine can be used. It is, of course, important to assure that ventilation is adequate so that there is no hypoxia or hypercarbia, since these can facilitate the development of arrhythmias as well as produce arrhythmias on their own.

The value of animal studies in determining the interaction of anesthetic agents and catecholamines can be demonstrated by the following observations. In studies of the dose of epinephrine required to produce arrhythmias during cyclopropane anesthesia, it was observed that in the cat the dose was 0.9 ug/kg (Katz and Bigger 1970). Thus, there is a good correlation between studies carried out in cats, dogs and man. However, human studies are the most important where it is feasible to perform them.

Up to now, we have discussed the subcutaneous injection of catecholamines. However, it is not uncommon in dentistry to make

intraosseous injection of catecholamines. Although, in general, small
amounts of local anesthetic and catecholamines are injected in dentistry,
the amounts used are sufficient to cause cardiovascular changes. For
example, Lilienthal and Reynolds (1975) studied intraosseous injection of
0.9 ml of 2% lidocaine with 1:80,000 epinephrine. This is a total dose of
epinephrine of 11.25 ug. They found that this increased heart rate and
blood pressure and produced palpitations and a sensation of a tight chest.
These cardiovascular signs and symptoms were not observed when the same
amounts of epinephrine and lidocaine were injected subcutaneously.

There have been numerous studies of the mechanism by which adrenergic
agents produce cardiac arrhythmias in the presence of halogenated hydrocarbons. Among the more important factors involved are the increase in
blood pressure and the increase in heart rate (Dresel et al. 1960, Vick
1966, Moe et al. 1948, Murphy et al. 1949, Katz 1965, Zink et al. 1975).
It has been well established in pharmacologic experiments that if the
heart rate increase is prevented or the increase in arterial pressure is
prevented that the arrhythmia threshold is increased. Since the injection
of a pharmacologic agent raises the question that in addition to the
prevention of the heart rate or blood pressure response, there may have
been an additional pharmacologic effect on the arrhythmia, the role of
blood pressure and heart rate has been studied with changes in these
parameters being prevented by mechanical means. A buffer bottle can be
used to prevent pressure changes and the heart rate can be controlled by
crushing the SA node and pacing the heart. In these kinds of experiments,
it has been observed that arrhythmias decreased in frequency or were
abolished by the lowering of blood pressure or by decreasing the heart
rate.

An interesting study of the catecholamines-anesthetic arrhythmias
was carried out by Miletich et al. (1978). They studied epinephrine
sensitivity in fasted and non-fasted rats. The arrhythmia threshold in
non-fasted rats was 10.9 ug/kg of epinephrine. In rats fasted 12, 24, and
48 hours, the arrhythmias threshold during halothane anesthesia was 5.5,
2.2 and 2.25 ug/kg. They also observed that the infusion of a 10% fatty
acid emulsion increased the epinephrine arrhythmia threshold. They
raised the question that fasting might cause a shift from a mixed
carbohydrate and lipid to a predominantly lipid metabolic response and
that this might render the heart more susceptible to arrhythmias. They

attempted to support this concept by pointing out that in patients with myocardial infarction, an elevated level of free fatty acid correlated with a higher frequency of arrhythmias. While these results of Miletich et al. are preliminary in nature, they raise many interesting questions concerning the implications of patients being fasted overnight.

REFLEX ARRHYTHMIAS

Cardiac arrhythmias are well-known to be reflexly initiated (Katz and Bigger 1970). The afferent limbs of the reflex may be activated by stimulation of the pharynx or trachea, traction on intra-abdominal or intrathoracic structures, manipulation of extraocular muscles and carotid sinus stimulation. The efferent limb of the reflex may be sympathetic and mediated by norepinephrine, epinephrine or may be parasympathetic and mediated by acetylcholine. Various combinations of sympathetic and parasympathetic stimulation and/or inhibition are possible. It is not possible to state in any given case what the net result may be. However, where the net result is either a relative or absolute increase in sympathetic activity, one may expect tachycardia, hypertension and cardiac arrhythmias. An example is tracheal intubation. On the other hand, when the net response is a relative or absolute increase in parasympathetic activity, bradycardia, hypotension and cardiac arrhythmias may be seen. A typical example of this is the oculo-cardiac reflex.

Depending upon the study quoted, the incidence of arrhythmias during tracheal intubation varies from 0-90% (Katz and Bigger 1970). These differences are probably explainable by variations in conditions of the study, the agents which the patient had been given prior to induction, the definition of arrhythmia and the method of recording and analyzing the arrhythmias. Suffice it to say that arrhythmias can be observed during intratracheal intubation and that these are usually associated with a relative sympathetic predominance. These arrhythmias are usually brief in duration and treatment is not necessary. The oculocardiac reflex or, more properly, the trigeminovagal reflex (defined in terms of the afferent and efferent limbs) is well-recognized. Traction on the extraocular muscles or pressure on the eyeball can provoke this reflex, which consists of bradycardia, hypotension and cardiac arrhythmias. The incidence of this reflex has been reported to range anywhere from 30-87% (Katz and Bigger 1970). Although the injection of atropine to block the efferent limb or retrobulbar block to prevent the afferent limb has been reported to be successful in several studies, we do not believe that these treatments should be routinely used for the following reasons: it is possible to elicit the reflex by doing a retrobulbar block. Furthermore, Berliner (1963) felt that the risk of complication in retrobulbar block was greater than the risk of arrhythmias. Intravenous atropine, although effective, can itself produce cardiac arrhythmias. Both Mendelblatt et al. (1962) and Pontinen (1966) found that although atropine reduced the incidence of arrhythmias, those arrhythmias which did occur were much more serious. In a study by Schwartz (1971) of almost 200 patients, he concluded that although retrobulbar block and atropine decreased the incidence of oculo-cardiac reflex by approximately 60%, the arrhythmias he observed with atropine were more severe and long-lasting than those in the untreated patients. He suggested, and it has been our practice even since then, to not treat the oculocardiac reflex prophylactically. Approximately 15 years of experience with this policy has led us to conclude that this is a worthwhile way of handling the problem. We currently monitor the electrocardiogram and if an arrhythmia appears and persists, the surgeon is asked to stop the manipulation temporarily. The arrhythmia disappears and with a more gentle handling of the eye it does not reappear.

HYPO AND HYPERKALEMIA

Both hypokalemia and hyperkalemia are capable of producing cardiac arrhythmias. Hypokalemia may occur with (1) renal dialysis; (2) anorexia, nausea, vomiting, diarrhea, intestinal obstruction, fistula with drainage of enteric fluid, nasogastric suction, prolonged parential feeding without adequate potassium supplementation; (3) familial periodic paralysis; (4) elevated levels of aldosterone; (5) diuretic therapy with thiazide, ethacrynic acid, furosemide, carbonic anhydrase inhibitors, and mercurial diuretics (Katz and Bigger 1970). Not infrequently, patients with these problems are scheduled for operations. It is important to raise the potassium to a satisfactory level before proceeding. Although we prefer to raise the potassium to 3.5 mEq/L, we frequently will proceed when the potassium has been raised to and is stabilized at 3.0 mEq/L. We point out the word "stabilize". If one is dealing with a hypokalemic patient and potassium is infused, it is fairly easy to raise the potassium to 3.0 mEq/L or greater transiently. However, if one continues to monitor the patient's potassium, it is not uncommon for the potassium to vary markedly and be quite low several hours after the infusion was given. Therefore, where possible, we prefer to stabilize the potassium at a level of 3.0 or greater over a period of 48 hours.

Hyperkalemia may also produce arrhythmias. This can be seen with (1) adrenal cortical insufficiency, (2) untreated diabetic acidosis, (3) renal disease, (4) sickle cell anemia, (5) multiple transfusions of stored blood, (6) diuretic therapy with aldactone or triamterine, (7) injection of succinylcholine in patients with burns, massive trauma, spinal cord injury, hemiplegia or paraplegia (Katz and Bigger 1970).

CYSTOSCOPY ARRHYTHMIAS

Kimbrough et al. (1975) observed that cardiac arrhythmias were not uncommon with cystoscopy. In a study of 69 men undergoing 191 cystoscopies, there were 36 patients with heart disease and 33 patients without heart disease. Ectopic beats, ventricular and supraventricular, occurred in 76% of the patients with heart disease and only 16% of those without heart disease. In patients who received general anesthesia, epidural anesthesia, or local lidocaine, frequency of ventricular ectopics was 8%, 14% and 49%, respectively, while there were no differences in supraventricular beats in these three groups. This study, along with others quoted previously, refute the widespread belief (particularly among internists) that local anesthesia is the cure for all operative problems in patients with heart disease.

RBB AND LAD

The combination of right bundle branch block and left axis deviation (RBB and LAD) occurs in 1% of patients. The question arises whether patients with right bundle branch block plus left axis deviation (presumably due to left anterior hemiblock or left anterior fasicle block) require the placement of a prophylactic pacemaker in case they go on to develop complete heart block during operation. DePascale and Bruno (1976) pointed out that the reason for the frequency of this combination is because the right bundle branch and the anterior fasicle of the left bundle branch are both supplied by the septal branch of the left anterior descending coronary. They also pointed out that RBB and LAD was

associated with a significant myocardial disease. In 27 patients with
this combination who underwent anesthesia, heart block did not develop
in any of the patients (Rooney et al. 1967). In 83 patients followed by
DePasquale and Bruno, complete heart block was seen in only 2 during
cumulative observation period of 262 patients years. Thus, it seems
reasonable to conclude that routine placement of a pacemaker in these
patients is not necessary.

PSYCHOPHARMACOLOGIC AGENTS

    Psychopharmacologic drugs used to treat patients have frequently
caused difficulties with arrhythmias. The problem of patients receiving
monoamine oxidase (MAO) inhibitors and subsequently eating food with
large amounts of tyramine and the resulting hypertension and cardiac
arrhythmias is well-documented. Although MAO inhibitors are being used
less frequently than in the past, a substantial number of patients are
on these drugs and one should remember that vasopressors which release
catecholamines and which are normally rapidly destroyed by monoamine
oxidase will pose problems. More commonly used than MAO inhibitors are
the tricyclic antidepressant agents. These post a threat for two reasons:
the tricyclic antidepressant agents block the reuptake of catecholamines
and therefore result in an increased circulating level of catecholamines.
Thus, patients on tricyclic antidepressants should receive smaller amounts
of catecholamines than normal, since they will overreact to these agents.
They should also receive smaller doses of drugs which will release
catecholamines in order to avoid severe hypertension and cardiac
arrhythmias. The second problem of the tricyclic and antidepressants
with which the anesthesiologist may have to deal involves their being used
in suicide attempts. In a study by Serafimovski et al. (9175) of 68 patients
with tricyclic antidepressant poisoning, 57 (84%) had severe electrocardiographic abnormalities. Another problem in treating these patients
stems from the anticholinergic belladonna-like action of the tricyclic
antidepressant, which may compound the arrhythmia problem and also
produce confusion and delirium. Brown (1976) has studied the mechanism
of arrhythmia induction with tricyclic antidepressants in the dog and has
compared a variety of methods of treating patients and animals with an
overdose of tricyclic antidepressants. He concluded that alkalinization
was the most effective method of treating the arrhythmias. Usually,

patients and animals with an overdose of tricyclic antidepressants had
a lowered pH, in the 7.17 to 7.27 range. The administration of 0.5-2
mEq/L of sodium bicarbonate was found to be the safest and most effective
treatment. If supplementary treatment was required, physostigmine was
the best additional agent to use, because the physostigmine not only had
a good antiarrhythmic effect, but also because it reversed the confusion
and delirium produced by the anticholinergic action of the tricyclic
antidepressant. This work confirms our own observations on the use of
physostigmines in the treatment of tricyclic antidepressant poisoning
(Katz and Katz 1972). It is interesting that we originally reported this
observation in 1971.

Another drug used in psychiatry which may produce problems is
lithium, which is commonly used in the treatment of depression. Wilson
et al. (1976), Targedahl and Gau (1972) and Tseng (1971) demonstrated
that lithium is capable of producing t-wave changes, sinus node block,
myocarditis, and ventricular arrhythmias. Thus, one should do a careful
history in patients presented for operation to determine whether a
patient is receiving psychotherapeutic agents, which may make them more
prone to the development of cardiac arrhythmias.

SUBARACHNOID HEMORRHAGE

Subarachnoid hemorrhage may cause centrally induced cardiac
arrhythmias. The sympathetic nature of this arrhythmia was shown by
Grossman (1976) who reported that left stellate ganglion block could
abolish cardiac arrhythmias in a patient with subarachnoid hemorrhage.
Studies in animals in our own laboratories demonstrated that stimulation
of the right stellate ganglion in the dog produced tachycardia, while
stimulation of the left stellate ganglion was more likely to produce
arrhythmias. This observation fits well with the efficacy of left
stellate ganglion block in abolishing centrally induced arrhythmias,
presumably due to increased sympathetic outflow following the subarachnoid hemorrhage.

INSECT VENOM ARRHYTHMIAS

An unusual cause of cardiac arrhythmia is following the sting of
either the yellow scorpion or the black widow spider (Weitzman et al.
1977). The effect of the venom on the autonomic nervous system results

in increased sympathetic discharge and an increased level of catecholamines. Weitzman et al. (1977) were able to document the increase level of urinary catecholamines; thus, these arrhythmias can be treated with beta adrenergic blockade.

MUSCLE RELAXANT INDUCED ARRHYTHMIAS

It has been known since 1958 (Moncrief) that the use of succinylcholine in burn patients may be dangerous. Since that time there have been numerous articles reporting cardiac arrhythmia and arrest in burn patients receiving succinylcholine. It was not until 1967 that Tolmie et al. demonstrated that hyperkalemia was the mechanism responsible for the cardiac problems. They were able to demonstrate a maximum rise in serum potassium of 8 mEq/L. Since then, many workers, including Mazze and Dunbar (1968), Weintraub et al. (1969), Birch et al. (1969) and Mazze et al. (1969) ave reported hyperkalemia not only in burn patients, but in patients with massive trauma who received succinylcholine. An increase in serum potassium in patients with tetanus who received succinylcholine was also reported by Roth and Wuthrich (1969). Cooperman et al. (1970) reported that hyperkalemia following succinylcholine may occur in patients with neurological disorders. They observed such responses in patients with paraplegia following spinal cord trauma, hemiperesis, multiple sclerosis, muscular dystrophy and cerebrovascular accidents. Others have reported succinylcholine-induced hyperkalemia in patients with paraplegia due to spinal cord injury (Stone et al. 1970) and in the Guillian-Bare Syndrome (Beach et al. 1971) as well as in patients with peripheral nerve injuries (Tobey et al. 1972). Recently, a hyper-kalemic response to succinylcholine in a patient with encephalitis has been reported (Cowgill et al. 1974).

There is some controversy over the response of the patient with renal failure to succinylcholine. One position is that the rise in potassium following succinylcholine in patients with renal failure is dangerous and that a depolarizing relaxant should not be used. However, the vast majority of studies have come to different conclusions. It has been reported by Paton (1956) that the normal response to succinylcholine is an increase in potassium of 0.5 mEq/L. Similar results were reported by Stovener et al. (1972) and by Dhanaraj (1975). In studies by Koide and Waud (1972) and Miller et al. (1972), the succinylcholine-induced increase in serum potassium was no greater in patients with renal failure than in normal patients. Thus, the vast majority of people who have studied the subject feel that the use of succinylcholine is safe in these patients. One point of caution is necessary: It has been reported that in patients with renal failure who have received two doses of succinyl-choline, while the first dose did not elevate potassium, the second dose did produce a rise of 2.8 mEq/L. No untoward effects were noted. A similar greater rise after the second dose of succinylcholine compared with the first dose in patients with renal failure has been described by Powell (1970) and Koide and Waud (1972). Although a second dose or a third dose may produce a greater rise in potassium than normally seen after the first dose, the magnitude of rise is still smaller than that seen in patients with burns. Finally, in a recent paper, Powell and Miller (1975) reported that in 11 patients with renal failure three doses of succinylcholine did not produce increases in potassium greater than 0.6 mEq/L. A reasonable conclusion would be that the evidence at this point suggests that the use of succinylcholine is safe in patients with renal failure.

One important observation is that in patients with burns, there is a period of time during which the patient is at greater risk of develop-ment of hyperkalemia than at other times. In general, it was believed that the susceptibility to succinylcholine-induced hyperthermia was from the 20th to the 60th post-burn day. However, the period of risk has been found to extend beyond these times. Furthermore, the period of risk with other disorders is not identical to that observed in burn patients. For example, Mazze et al. (1969) found that in patients with massive trauma, the danger period extended from three weeks until the lesion was covered by skin. Cooperman et al. (1970) reported that the danger period following spinal cord injury was usually less than 6 months, but could be longer where there was progressive neurological disease. Tobie et al. (1972), who studied lower motor neuron injuries, found the danger period a half a year or more. In view of the marked variation in time period during which a patient may develop hyperkalemia in response to succinylcholine, it would be wise in most situations in which there is any doubt to avoid the use of succinylcholine.

In an elegant group of studies, Gronert and associates (Gronert and Theye 1971), Gronert, Lambert and Theye 1973) studied potassium flux after succinylcholine injection in normal, immobilized, paraplegic and denervated canine muscles. The greatest potassium flux occurred in the denervated muscles, the next greatest in paraplegic muscles, and the smallest in immobilized muscles. These workers observed that a small dose of non-depolarizing relaxant diminished the hyperkalemic response, but did not block it. It is, therefore, clinically important to remember that the prior injection of a small dose of non-depolarizer will not completely inhibit the succinylcholine-induced hyperkalemia in burn and trauma patients and, therefore, it would seem wiser to avoid succinylcholine.

Bradycardia following injection of succinylcholine was reported shortly after its introduction into clinical practice. Phillips in 1954 reported a decrease in pulse rate to 40 beats per minute. Leigh et al. in 1957 reported that the intravenous injection of succinylcholine in infants and children sometimes produces bradycardia. Numerous studies since that time have reported bradycardia, sinus arrest, superventricular and ventricular arrhythmias following repeated intravenous injection of succinylcholine in infants, children and adults anesthetized with nitrous oxide, trichloroethylene, ether, halothane and cyclopropane. It is important to remember that the response in children and adults differs. Bradycardia in children is often seen following the first dose of succinylcholine, while in the adult this is rarely observed. In the adult, bradycardia is commonly seen following a second dose of succinylcholine, particularly when the interval between the two doses is five minutes. Under these circumstances, bradycardia occurs in 80% or more of adults. There have been a number of studies of the mechanism of bradycardia following succinylcholine. In general, it appears that the bradycardia and arrhythmias are due to stimulation of both the sympathetic and parasympathetic nervous systems. In any given individual depending upon the age, the anesthetic agent and the circumstances of injection, one may get a predominance of sympathetic or parasympathetic stimulation. Schoenstadt and Whitcher (1963) studied five patients who received repeated injections of succinylcholine. There were no arrhythmias in five patients in whom anesthesia was induced with thiopental and maintained with halothane, but there were arrhythmias in five patients in whom anesthesia was induced and maintained with halothane. Furthermore, three of the patients in the latter group, after injection of thiopental no

longer developed arrhythmias with repeated injections of succinylcholine.
These workers also found that patients who received hexafluorenine did
not develop arrhythmias after succinylcholine. Furthermore, patients
given acetylcholine did not develop arrhythmias after a second dose of
acetylcholine. However, four out of five patients given succinylcholine
after acetylcholine developed bradycardia or asystole. These results
suggest that choline, which is produced by the hydrolysis of succinylcholine or acetylcholine sensitizes patients to subsequent doses of
succinylcholine, but not acetylcholine. Thus, choline is the sensitizer,
but succinylcholine is required to produce the arrhythmia.

In other studies of the site of action of succinylcholine bradycardia,
Mathias and Evans Prosser (1968) injected small amounts of succinylcholine
directly into the common carotid artery and, therefore, presumably into
the pressor receptors of the carotid sinus. In more than one-third of the
patients an immediate slowing of the heart was observed. It is, therefore, postulated that succinylcholine was able to stimulate peripheral
sensory receptors (such as carotid sinus baroreceptors) and produce
reflex bradycardia. It is well-known that acetylcholine, structurally
similar to succinylcholine, has a stimulant action on pressor receptors
and other sensory receptors.

The bradycardia produced by repeated doses of succinylcholine can be
blocked by hexafluorenium and by small doses of non-depolarizing agents.
Although it is possible to block the response, one wonders whether it was
worth it. In our own studies of repeated doses of succinylcholine,
although bradycardia does occur following a second dose given five minutes
after an initial dose, the bradycardia has always been self-limiting and
brief in duration. Thus, when the need for a second dose of succinylcholine for intratracheal intubation is necessary, it seems reasonable
to carefully watch the EKG and be prepared to inject atropine if
necessary. However, in our experience, it has never been necessary to
inject atropine, since the bradycardia has always disappeared spontaneously
in a brief period of time, always less than one minute.

Cardiac arrhythmias following the injection of gallamine were
reported in patients anesthetized with cyclopropane by Walts and
Prescott (1965). Tachycardia and hypertension following gallamine have
long been known. In general, it appears likely that the major mechanism
responsible for the tachycardia, hypertension and arrhythmia is vagal

blockade. There is some dispute as to whether these effects may also
be due to the release of catecholamines from cardiac adrenergic nerves.
It seems that although it is possible in animals to demonstrate catecholamine release by gallamine (Brown and Crout 1970) this does not
appear to occur in man (Reitan et al. 1973). Recently, pancuronium has
been demonstrated to be capable under certain circumstances of increasing
blood pressure and heart rate and possibly producing cardiac arrhythmias.
This effect seems to be due to a weak vagal blocking action of pancuronium,
an action that is much less than that seen with gallamine (in equipotent
neuromuscular blocking doses).

SICK SINUS SYNDROME (SSS)

The sick sinus syndrome consists of sinus bradycardia or arrest with
or without associated superventricular tachycardia. As originally defined
by Ferrer (1968) it may include sinus bradycardia, sinus arrest, sinoatrial block, alternating bradyarrhythmias, tachyarrhythmias, and carotid
hypersensitivity. The disease is sometimes referred to as the bradytachyarrhythmia syndrome in patients who have alternating bradycardia and
tachycardia. The subject has been reviewed by Scarpa (1976). In general,
the mechanism is due to a disoredered impulse generation in the sinus
node or impaired conduction from the sinus node into the atrium. The
anatomy of the sinus node is such that the primary blood supply is almost
always a single vessel which arises from the proximal few centimeters of
the right coronary artery in 55% of cases, and the proximal few milli-
meters of the left circumflex artery in 45%. It should be remembered
that the same artery supplies most of the atria and that this disease
has also been referred to as the sick sinus and ailing atrium. Many
cases of the SSS occurred in patients with coronary artery disease. In
the series of 74 patients studied by Moss and Davis (1974), in 51 there
was associated coronary artery disease, and idiopathic heart disease
accounted for 34% of their cases. The remainder had hypertension,
rheumatic heart disease, congenital heart disease, and cardiomyopathy.
Furthermore, digitalis, quinidine, procaine amide and propranolol can all
produce an ECG and clinical picture of the sick sinus syndrome.

There is no sex preponderance, with equal numbers of men and women
affected. Although the peak incidence is in the 7th decade, the SSS also
occurs in children. The brain, heart and kidney are the organs most

affected and which give signs and symptoms. Moss and Davis (1974) reported that 48% of their patients with bradytachyarrhythmias had cerebral manifestations including syncopy, near syncopy and dizziness. Their review of the literature revealed that 75% of the reported cases had these symptoms, as did 40 of 56 reported by Rubinstein et al (1972). Because of the changing atrial pattern with bradytachyarrhythmias, embolization is not uncommon, and occurred in 8 of 33 of the patients reported by Rubinstein et al. (1972). In the Moss and Davis study (1974), 25 of 74 patients had syncopy. The second most prominent organ producing symptoms of the SSS is the heart itself. These include palpitations, angina, and manifestations of congestive heart disease. These may be due to tachycardia as well as failure of the heart to develop tachycardia under an appropriate stimulus. Unexplained episodes of pulmonary edema, ventricular failure or angina may be the result of the arrhythmias of the SSS.

The most frequent single arrhythmia in the SSS is sinus bradycardia, reported in 76% of patients of Moss and Davis (1974). A variety of other superventricular arrhythmias occur, such as sinus arrest, junctional bradycardia, wandering pacemaker, superventricular ectopic beats, intermittent sinus arrest. The occurrence of ventricular arrhythmias in SSS is unusual, occurring in only 10% of the patients of Moss and Davis (1974) and none of the patients of Rubinstein et al. (1972). The tachycardia arrhythmias of the bradytachyarrhythmia syndrome are mainly superventricular.

The diagnosis comes from the history, which includes palpitations, angina and symptoms of congestive failure, as well as syncopy. Physical exam is not helpful, but the ECG is very important. Holter monitoring has been very valuable in these patients. Episodic bradytachyarrhythmias as well as other arrhythmias can be documented. When symptoms and arrhythmias concur with Holter monitoring, the diagnosis is almost assured. It should be remembered when attempting to make a diagnosis that no clearcut cardiac etiology may be seen. This was the case in 25 of 56 patients studied by Rubinstein et al. (1972).

A diagnostic provocative test is the valsalva maneuver. Patients with SSS have a normal blood pressure response to valsalva, but there is little or no change in pulse rate. Also, they do not respond to atropine. Ferrer states that if 1-2 mg of IV atropine does not increase sinus bradycardia to a rate exceeding 90 per min, and if after atropine sinus node recovery time remains prolonged after overdrive, the diagnosis is made. The most valuable provocative test in SSS is atrial pacing. Pacing starts at 90 beats per min and increases to 150. At the end of the period, the pacing is terminated and the interval from the last pacing stimulus to the onset of the next t-waves is measured. This represents the sinus node recovery time. An even better concept is that of the corrective sinus node recovery time, which is the difference between the recovery interval following tachypacing and the average resting interval.

Patients may be divided into those who have major or minor syndromes. Major includes cerebral, coronary or low output problems. Minor includes ankle enema, subjective palpitations and an uncomfortable awareness of a slow, rapid or irregular heartbeat. Patients with minor symptoms may be managed with reassurance. Those with major symptoms require therapy. Pacemaker therapy remains the foundation of the treatment. In general, belladonna drugs to treat bradycardia are ineffective. In the study of Rubinstein et al. (1972), belladonna alkaloids did not speed the sinus rate on 14 occasions, and in 4 cases, patients were worse because of the side effect. There was induction of tachyarrhythmia in 2. In only 2 patients with bradycardia did chronic administration of atropine seem to help. Similarly, sympathomimetic amines were ineffective in 11 cases, and 5 patients were worse because of their side effects or induction of tachyarrhythmia. Pacing was employed in 23 of 56 patients, permanent in 18 and temporary in 5. This was the most successful therapy. A special value of pacemaker implantation is that it permits the addition of digitalis or propranolol without the feat of aggravating the bradycardia. Thus, in most cases, permanent ventricular pacing remains the therapy of choice. If there are no AV conduction disturbances, atrial pacing may be considered, but more likely ventricular pacemakers will be necessary. In the study of Rubinstein, six of the 56 patients studied died during an average following period of seven years. However, in only one case was the death related to the SSS.

ANTI-ARRHYTHMIC AGENTS

There are a number of drugs commonly used for the control of arrhythmias, including procaine amide, quinidine, propranolol, diphenylhydantoin (dilantin) and lidocaine. Although these drugs can be effective in many patients, drug therapy is rarely necessary. If one

reviews the above discussion, it should be obvious that in the vast
majority of cases, the arrhythmia can best be treated by eliminating the
cause, i.e., lowering the concentration of anesthetic agent, decreasing
Pco_2 to normal, avoiding hypoxia, or avoiding the injection of excessive
amounts of catecholamines. Therefore, in the vast majority of cases, an
anti-arrhythmic agent is not needed. In a few cases, lidocaine, 1-2 mg/kg
may be given. The circumstances under which this may be useful is where
the cause of the arrhythmia is not immediately obvious and one needs to
buy time, i.e., 10-20 minutes to review the anesthetic management,
surgical manipulation and make appropriate changes. In these
circumstances, the injection of lidocaine is reasonable. In rare
special circumstances, agents such as diphenyhydantoin or propranolol
may be of value. For those interested in these agents, their use has been
previously reviewed. (Katz and Bigger, 1970)

CONCLUSIONS
1. Arrhythmias frequently are seen even in the well-managed patient
   undergoing anesthesia and surgery. However, drug treatment is
   rarely required.
2. With less than optimal anesthetic management, cardiac arrhythmias
   can be a warning that the patient is in physiologic or pharmacologic distress and that rapid remedial action is necessary.
   Thus, the onset of arrhythmia should initiate an immediate
   evaluation of anesthetic management and surgical events.
3. In general, slow super-ventricular rhythm, such as atrial rhythm,
   AV junctional rhythm and wandering pacemaker are benign and do not
   require treatment. However, ventricular arrhythmias should be
   considered a sign of serious physiological derangement until
   proven otherwise.
4. The electrocardiographic appearance of an arrhythmia does not
   necessarily identify the mechanism responsible for the arrhythmia
   or the circulatory effect of the arrhythmia.
5. Most arrhythmias can be explained in terms of an autonomic nervous
   system imbalance. Sympathetic predominance may occur by an increase
   in sympathetic activity or a decrease in parasympathetic activity.
   Similarly, parasympathetic predominance may be either absolute
   or relative.

6. Arrhythmias may be due not only to changes occurring primarily in the heart, but also to primary changes in the central nervous system or in the periphery.

ABSTRACT

This paper reaches the following conclusions:

1. Arrhythmias frequently are seen even in the well-managed patient undergoing anesthesia and surgery. However, drug treatment is rarely required.

2. With less than optimal anesthetic management, cardiac arrhythmias can be a warning that the patient is in physiologic or pharmacologic distress and that rapid remedial action is necessary. Thus, the onset of arrhythmia should initiate an immediate evaluation of anesthetic management and surgical events.

3. In general, slow super-ventricular rhythm, such as atrial rhythm, AV junctional rhythm and wandering pacemaker are benign and do not require treatment. However, ventricular arrhythmias should be considered a sign of serious physiological derangement until proven otherwise.

4. The electrocardiographic appearance of an arrhythmia does not necessarily identify the mechansim responsible for the arrhythmia or the circulator effect of the arrhythmia.

5. Most arrhythmias can be explained in terms of an autonomic nervous system imbalance. Sympathetic predominance may occur by an increase in sympathetic activity or a decrease in parasympathetic activity. Similarly, parasympathetic predominance may be either absolute or relative.

6. Arrhythmias may be due not only to changes occurring primarily in the heart, but also to primary changes in the central nervous system or in the periphery.

160

REFERENCES

1. Levy AG, Lewis T. Heart irregularities resulting from the inhalation of low perecentages of chloroform vapour and their relationship to ventricular fibbrilation. Heart 1911-12;3:99.
2. Levy AG. Sudden death under light chloroform anesthesia. J Physiol 1911;42:3.
3. Dodd RB, Sims WA, Bone DJ. Cardiac arrhythmias observed during anesthesia. Surgery 1962;51:440.
4. Reinikainen M, Pontinen P. On cardiac arrhythmias during anesthesia and surgery. Acta Med Scand 1966;180: suppl. 457.
5. Kuner J, Enescu V, Utsu F, Boszormenyi E, Bernstein H, Corday E. Cardiac arrhythmias during anesthesia. Dis Chest 1967;52:580.
6. Vanik PE, Davis HS. Cardiac arrhythmias during halothane anesthesia. Anesth Analg 1968;47:299.
7. Katz RL, Bigger JT Jr. Cardiac arrhythmias during anesthesia and operation. Anesthesiology 1970;33:193.
8. Hughes CL, Leach JK, Allen RE, Lambson GO. Cardiac arrhythmias during oral surgery with local anesthesia. J Amer Dent Ass 1966; 73:1095.
9. Stephen CR, North WC. Halopropane: A clinical evaluation. Anesthesiology 1964;25:600.
10. Katz RL. Antiarrhythmic and neuromuscular effects of QX-527 in man. Acta Anaesth Scand 1965;9:73.
11. Artusio JF, Poznak AV, Weingram J, Sohn YJ. Teflurane, a non-explosive gas for clinical anesthesia. Anesth Analg 1967;46:657.
12. Lurie AA, Jones RE, Linde HW, Price ML, Kripps RD, Price HL. Cyclopropane anesthesia: Cardiac rate and rhythm during steady levels of cyclopropane anesthesia at normal and elevated end-expiratory, carbon dioxide tensions. Anesthesiology 1958;19:457.
13. Waters RM, Orth OS, Gillespie NA. Trichloroethylene anesthesia and cardiac rhythm. Anesthesiology 1943;4:1.
14. Katz RL. Neural factors affecting cardiac arrhythmias induced by halopropane. J Pharmacol Exp Ther 1966;152:88.
15. Beattie J, Brow GR, Long CNH. The hypothalamus and the sympathetic nervous system. Proc Ass Res Nerv Dis 1928;9:249.
16. Price HL, Lurie AA, Jones RE, Price ML, Linde HW. Cyclopropane anesthesia: Epinephrine and norepinephrine in initiation of ventricular arrhythmias by carbon dioxide inhalation. Anesthesiology 1958;19:619.
17. Black GW, Linde HW, Dripps RD, Price HL. Circulatory changes accompanying respiratory acidosis during halothane (Fluothane) anesthesia in man. Brit J Anaes 1959;31:238.
17a. Eikard B, Skovsted P. Effects of respiratory acidosis on the arrhythmia threshold during fluroxene and halothane anesthesia. Acta Anaesth Scand 1975;19:120.
18. Katz RL, Epstein RA. The interaction of anesthetic agents and adrenergic drugs to produce cardiac arrhythmias. Anesthesiology 1968;29:763.
19. Katz RL, Lord CO, Evans KE. Anesthetic-dopamine cardiac arrhythmias and their prevention by beta adrenergic blockade. J Pharmacol Exp Ther 1967;158:40.

20. Zahed B, Miletich DJ, Ivankovich AD, Albrecht RF, Tayooka ET. Arrhythmic doses of epinephrine and dopamine during halothane, enflurane, methoxyflurane and fluroxene anesthesia in goats. Anesth and Analg 1977;56:207.
21. Vidouse JP. Intravenous perfusion of adrenalin during enflurane anesthesia. Acta Anaesth Belgica 1975;2-3:94.
22. Lippmann M, Reisner LS. Epinephrine injection with enflurane anesthesia: Incidence of cardiac arrhythmias. Anesth and Analg 1974;53:886.
23. Konchigeri HN, Shaker MH, Winnie AP. Effect of epinephrine during enflurane anesthesia. Anesth and Analg 1974;53:894.
24. Suzuki A, Yanai K, Taki K. Comparison of epinephrine injection during enflurane and halothane anesthesia. Jap J Anesth 1976;25:490.
25. Conner JR, Miller JD, Katz RL. Isoflurane anesthesia for pheochromocytoma: A case report. Anes and Analg 1975;54 (4):419.
26. Katz RL, Wolf CE. Pheochromocytoma. In: Highlights of Clinical Anesthesiology. Mark LC, Ngai SG. eds. New York: Harper and Row, 1971:55-65.
27. Milgrave AP. Epinephrine with halothane in children. Canad Anesth Soc J 1970;17:256.
28. Lilienthal B, Reynolds AK. Cardiovascular responses to intraosseous injections containing catecholamines. Oral Surg 1975;40:574.
29. Dresel PE, MacCannell KL, Niekerson M. Cardiac arrhythmias induced by minimal doses of epinephrine in cyclopropane anesthetized dogs. Circ Res 1960;8:948.
30. Vick RL. Effects of altered heart rate on chloroform-epinephrine cardiac arrhythmias. Circ Res 1966;18:316.
31. Moe GK, Malton SD, Rennick BR, Freyburger WA. The role of arterial pressure in the induction of idioventricular rhythms under cyclopropane anesthesia. J Pharmacol Exp Ther 1948;94:319.
32. Murphy Q, Crumpton CW, Meek WJ. The effect of blood pressure rise on the production of cyclopropane-epinephrine induced cardiac arrhythmias. Anesthesiology 1949;10:416.
33. Katz RL. The effect of alpha and beta adrenergic blocking agents on cyclopropane-catecholamine cardiac arrhythmias. Anesthesiology 1965;26:289.
34. Zink J, Sasyniuk BI, Dresel PE. Halothane-epinephrine-induced cardiac arrhythmias and the role of heart rate. Anesthesiology 1975;43:548.
35. Miletick DJ, Abrecht RF, Seals C. Influence of fasting on epinephrine arrhythmias during halothane anesthesia. Anesthesiology 1978. In press.
36. Berler DK. The oculocardiac reflex. Amer J Opthal 1963;56:954.
37. Mendelblatt FJ, Kirsch RE, Lemberg L. Preventing the oculocardiac reflex. Amer J Ophthal 1962;53:506.
38. Pontinen PJ. The importance of the oculocardiac reflex during ocular surgery. Acta Ophthal 1966, suppl. 86.
39. Schwartz H. Oculocardiac reflex: Is prophylaxis necessary? Highlights of Clinical Anesthesiology. Mark LC, Ngai SH, eds. New York: Harper and Row, 1971:11.
40. Kimbrough HM, Crampton RS, Gillenivaler JY. Cardiac rhythm in men during cystoscopy. J Urol 1975;113:846.
41. DePasquale VP, Bruno MS. Natural history of combined right bundle branch block and left anterior hemiblock. Am J Med 1973;54:297.
42. Rooney SA, Goldiner PL, Musa E. Relationship of right bundle branch block and marked left axes deviation to complete heart block during general anesthesia. Anesthesiology 1976;44:64.

43. Serafimovski N, Thorball N, Asmussan I, Lunding M. Tricyclic anti-depressive poisoning with special reference to cardiac complications. Acta Anaesth Scand 1975, suppl 57:55.

44. Brown TCK. Tricyclic antidepressant overdosage: Experimental studies on the management of circulatory complications. Clin Toxicol 1976; 9:255.

45. Katz RL, Katz GJ. Surgical infiltration of pressure drugs and their interaction with volatile anesthetics. Brit J Anaes 1966;27:756.

46. Wilson JR, Kraus ES, Bailas MM, Rakita L. Reversible sinus-node abnormalities due to lithium carbonate therapy. Med Intel 1976;294: 1223.

47. Tengedhal TN, Gau GT. Myocardial irritability associated with lithium carbonate therapy. N Engl J Med 1972;287:867.

48. Tseng HL. Interstitial myocarditis probably related to lithium carbonate intoxication. Arch Pathol 1971;92:444.

49. Grossman MA. Cardiac arrhythmias in acute central nervous system disease. Arch Int Med 1976;136:203.

50. Weitzman S, Margules G, Lehmann E. Uncommon cardiovascular manifest-ations and high catecholamine levels due to "black widow" bite. Am Heart J 1977;93:89.

51. Moncrief JA. Complications of burns. Ann Surg 1958;147:443.

52. Tolmie JD, Joyce TH, Mitchell GD. Succinylcholine danger in the burned patient. Anesthesiology 1967;28:467.

53. Mazze RI, Dunbar RW. Intralingual succinylcholine administration in children: An alternative to intravenous and intramuscular routes? Anesth Analg Curr Res 1968;47:605.

54. Weintraub HD, Heisterkamp DV, Cooperman LH. Changes in plasma potassiur concentration after depolarizing blockers in anesthetized man. Br J Anaesth 1969;41:1048.

55. Birch AA Jr., Mitchell GD, Playford GA. Changes in plasma potassium response to succinylcholine following trauma. JAMA 1969;210:490.

56. Mazze RI, Escrue HM, Houston JR. Hyperkalemia and cardiovascular collapse following administration of succinylcholine to the trauma-tized patient. Anesthesiology 1969;31:540.

57. Roth F, Wuthrich H. The clinical importance of hyperkalemia following suxamethonium administration. Br J Anaesth 1969;41:311.

58. Cooperman LH, Strobel GE Jr, Kennell EM. Massive hyperkalemia after administration of succinylcholine. Anesthesiology 1970;32:161.

59. Stone WA, Beach TP, Hamelberg W. Succinylcholine-danger in the spinal-cord-injured patient. Anesthesiology 1970;32:168.

60. Beach TP, Stone WA, Hamelberg W. Circulatory collapse following succinylcholine: Report of a patient with diffuse lower motor neuron disease. Anesth Analg Curr Res 1971;50:431.

61. Tobey RE, Jacobsen PM, Kahle CT et al. The serum potassium response to muscle relaxants in neural injury. Anesthesiology 1972;37:332.

62. Cowgill DB, Mostello LA, Shapiro HM. Encephalitis and a hyperkalemic response to succinylcholine. Anesthesiology 1974;40:409.

63. Paton WDH. Mode of action of neuromuscular blocking agents. Brit J Anaesth 1956;28:490.

64. Stover J, Endressen R, Bjelke E. Suxamethonium hyperkalemia with different induction agents. Acta Anaesth Scand 1972;16:46.

65. Dhanaraj VJ, Narayanamurthy J, Sitadevi C, Mohan Rao K. A study of the changes in serum potassium concentration with suxamethonium using different anesthetic agents. Br J Anaesth 1975;47:516.

66. Koide M, Waud BE. Serum potassium concentrations after succinylcholine in patients with renal failure. Anesthesiology 1972;36:142.
67. Miller RD, Way WL, Hamilton WK, Layzer RB. Succinylcholine-induced hyperkalemia in patients with renal failure. Anesthesiology 1972; 36:138.
68. Powell JN. Suxamethonium-induced hyperkalemia in a uraemic patient. Br J Anaesth 1970;42:806.
69. Powell DR, Miller R. The effect of repeated doses of succinylcholine on serum potassium in patients with renal failure. Anesth Analg Curr Res 1975;54:746.
70. Gronert GA, Theye RA. Serum potassium changes after succinylcholine in swine with thermal trauma or sciatic nerve section. Can Anesth Soc J 1971;18:558.
71. Gronert GA, Lambert EH, Theye RA. The response of denervated skeletal muscle to succinylcholine. Anesthesiology 1973;39:13.
72. Phillips HS. Physiologic changes noted with the use of succinylcholine chloride as a muscle relaxant during endotracheal intubation. Anesth Analg 1954;33:165.
73. Leigh MD, McCoy DD, Belton MK, Lewis GB. Bradycardia following intravenous administration of succinylcholine chloride to infants and children. Anesthesiology 1957;18:698.
74. Schoenstadt DA, Whitcher CE. Observations on the mechanism of succinylcholine-induced cardiac arrhythmias. Anesthesiology 1963; 24:358.
75. Mathias JA, Evans-Prosser C. An investigation into the site of action of suxamethonium on cardiac rhythm. Proceedings of Fourth World Congress of Anesthesiologists, 1968, London, 1153.
76. Walts LF, Prescott FS. The effects of gallamine on cardiac rhythm during general anesthesia. Anesth Analg 1965;44:265.
77. Brown ER, Crout JR. The sympathomimetic effect of gallamine on the heart. Anesthesiology 1968;29:179.
78. Reitan JA, Fraser AI, Eisele JH. Lack of cardiac inotropic effects of gallamine in anesthetized man. Anesth Analg Curr Res 1973;52:974.
79. Ferrer MI. The sick sinus syndrome in atrial disease. JAMA 1968; 206:645.
80. Scarpa WJ. The sick sinus symdrome. Am Heart J 1976;92:648.
81. Moss AJ, Davis RJ. Brady-tachy syndrome. Prog Cardiovasc Dis 1974; 16:439.
82. Rubenstein J, Schulman C, Yurchak, Pavd De Sanctis R. Clinical spectrum of the sick sinus syndrome. Circulation 1972;46:5.

INVASIVE AND NON-INVASIVE MONITORING OF MYOCARDIAL ISCHEMIA DURING NON-CARDIAC SURGERY

Sebastian Reiz, MD, PhD.

Recently, the close association between intraoperative ischemia and post-operative myocardial infarction in patients after coronary artery bypass grafting (CABG) has been established (1). In patients with peripheral arterial disease, it is possible to predict postoperative ischemic insults to the heart from preoperative dipyridamole-thallium scintigraphy (2). As yet, there are however no studies on preoperative prediction of perioperative myocardial ischemia. Coronary angiography has revealed coronary artery disease (CAD) in more than 90% of patients with abdominal aortic aneurysms, claudication or carotid artery disease (3). Approximately 50% of these patients fullfilled the criteria for CABG. However, many have little or no cardiac symptoms because of their functional limitation and therefore do not come for CABG evaluation. The morbidity and mortality in cardiovascular complications remain at or above that reported for CABG (4). Consequently, a sensitive clinical indicator of myocardial ischemia to alert the anesthetist and allow him to respond promptly would appear to be the key to avoiding permanent consequences of ischemia, whatever the cause.

Ischemia following progressive narrowing of a coronary artery in the experimental animal produces wall motion abnormalities which precede ECG changes, lactate production, increase in filling pressure of the ventricle or global pump dysfunction (5). Thus, wall motion abnormality is the most sensitive indicator of ischemia under experimental conditions. Similar results have recently been documented in patients with CAD in whom areas of abnormal wall motion detected by 2-D echo-cardiography after dipyridamole coincided with angiographically demonstrable obstructions to the same territories (6). In the operating room, we still rely on electrocardiographic monitoring for the detection of myocardial ischemia, at best using paper recordings of the V5 and II leads. Special ST-segment monitors, which integrate the areas of multiple lead ST-segments have been developed to improve the sensitivity of ECG monitoring (7). In the last few years, some interesting reports on monitoring of wall motion have appeared in the litterature (8,9). The two techniques utilized are cardiokymography (CKG) and 2-D echo-cardiography. Since the latter technique is highly invasive, costly and cannot be introduced prior to induction of anesthesia, little documentation of its reliability exists. As yet, there are few,if any studies, in which the various techniques to detect myocardial ischemia perioperatively have been compared. The scope of this presentation is to present a summary of our most recent data from comparative studies of the ECG, CKG, myocardial lactate balance and the pulmonary capillary wedge pressure (PCWP) as indicators of perioperative myocardial ischemia in patients undergoing peripheral arterial revascularization.

ELECTROCARDIOGRAPHY VERSUS MYOCARDIAL LACTATE BALANCE.

Well-oxygenated myocardium is a lactate extractor; as oxygenation becomes deficient, myocardium produces lactate. When oxygen imbalance is regional rather than global, coronary sinus measurements may reflect this by a decrease in lactate extraction. Obviously, regional sampling is desirable to document the disparate myocardial nutrition. This may be accomplished by catheterizing the great cardiac vein (GCV) via the coronary sinus (CS). This vein drains most of the anterior wall, perfused by the left anterior descending coronary artery (LAD). The same area is monitored by the V2 to V5 leads of the 12 lead ECG.

We studied 26 patients with lactate production from the LAD territory. Twelve patients only (46%) had simultaneously appearing ECG abnormalitites, most commonly in their V5 lead (11 of 12 abnormal observations). These were defined as a depression or pseudonormalization of the ST-segment of 0.1 mV or greater measured 80 msec after the maximal R-wave. Fourteen patients demonstrated unchanged 12 lead ECG-s with the onset of myocardial lactate production (Fig 1).

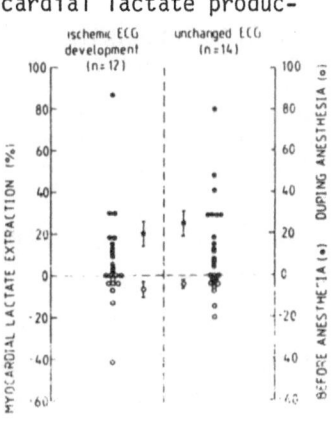

Fig 1. Change in myocardial lactate extraction in patients who developed simulataneous ECG abnormalities (left) compared with those in whom the ECG remained unchanged (right panel). Mean values of lactate extraction did not differ between groups. The 12 lead ECG had a 46% sensitivity to detect lactate production in the underlying region.

166

In another set of experiments, we studied the change in myocardial lactate extraction (sampling from the CS) occurring with development of ischemic
changes in the V5 lead. This lead has been reported abnormal in approximately
85% of ischemic episodes (10). Patients with a normal preoperative ECG and CAD
(n=13) were compared with patients without history of cardiovascular disease
(n=14). In the normal patients, induction of anesthesia did not produce any
change in myocardial lactate extraction. One of 35 measurements was associated
with a greater than 50% reduction of lactate extraction (Fig 2, right panel).
In the patients with CAD, non-ischemic ECG episodes were associated with unchanged lactate extraction and 2 observations only with greater than 50% reduction (Fig 2, left panel). When ischemic ECG changes were first observed, 26
of 28 measurements demonstrated a reduction of lactate extraction greater than
50%. Nine measurements only showed lactate production. Thus, lactate extraction
had to decrease by at least 50% before ECG changes were observed.

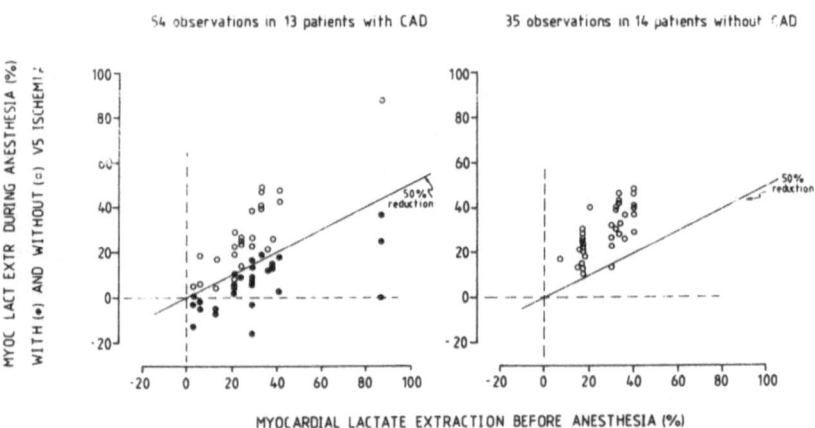

Fig 2. Relationship of coronary sinus lactate extraction before anesthesia to
lactate extraction during anesthesia in 13 patients who demonstrated ischemia
on ECG at least once during anesthesia and in 14 patients without CAD. Virtually all ECG changes were associated with reduction of greater than 50% in
lactate extraction. The data suggest that large decreases of lactate extraction may be indicative of regional ischemia during anesthesia.

CARDIOKYMOGRAPHY, ELECTROCARDIOGRAPHY AND LACTATE BALANCE.
    CKG has been used in conjunction with the standard exercise test as an
additional marker of ischemia (11,12). It records anterior wall motion via
changes in an electromagnetic field (Fig 4). A recent multicenter study has
documented a sensitivity and specificity significantly higher than the exercise

ECG and comparable to the thallium stress test (13). During anesthesia, the CKG has been shown to be highly sensitive in detecting periinduction ischemia among patients scheduled for CABG (8). We compared the ability of the CKG and ECG to detect a reduction of at least 50% in myocardial lactate extraction, using coronary sinus sampling. The results are shown in Fig 3 and Table 1 and demonstrate a significantly greater sensitivity but lesser specificity for the CKG.

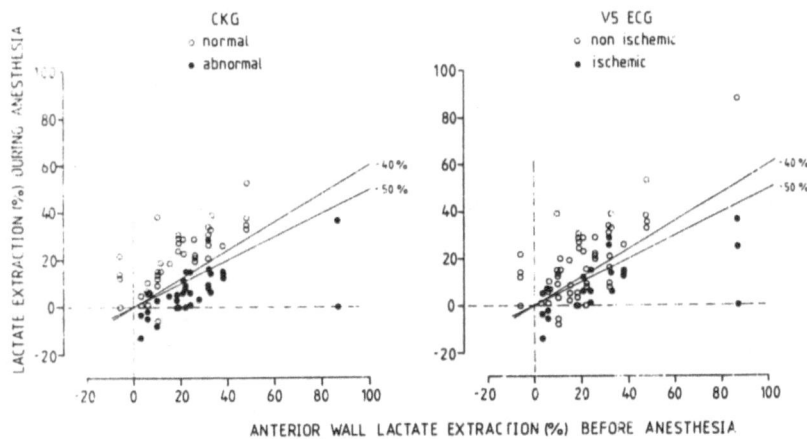

Fig 3. Comparison of the ability of the CKG (left) and the V5 ECG to detect changes in myocardial lactate extraction.

Table 1. Sensitivity and specificity of the CKG and the V5 ECG to detect a reduction in lactate extraction of 50% or greater.

	CKG	ECG	Concordant ECG & CKG
Sensitivity (%)	90	57	93
Specificity (%)	88	94	96

Non-interpretable CKG-s: 6.5% (discordant readings by 2 independent readers)

FILLING PRESSURE AND STROKE VOLUME USED AS INDICATORS OF ISCHEMIA.

In the last set of experiments, we studied 53 patients with CAD, scheduled to undergo peripheral arterial surgery with a wide variety of anesthetic agents and techniques. Simultaneous measurments and recordings of the 12 lead ECG, CKG, myocardial lactate balance (GCV sampling), stroke volume and PCWP/CVP were ob-

168

tained awake, during intubation, before onset of surgery and 10 and 30 min
post incision. A total of 261 data points were analyzed. Ischemia was defined
as one or more of the following criteria: 1) appearance of type II or III CKG
(Fig 4), 2) ECG changes defined as above and 3) myocardial lactate production.
The most striking finding in this study was the high incidence of abnormal CKG-s
recorded in 2/3 of the patients sometimes during anesthesia. Ischemic ECG-s
were recorded in 1/3 of the patients only. This incidence is in agreement with
previous studies in comparable patients (14).   A similar relationship between
the abnormal CKG-s and ECG-s was reported by Bellows et al (8). The total number
of intraoperative ischemic events and their mode of detection are outlined in
Table 2.

Table 2. Perioperative ischemic events; mode of diagnosis and relation to insult.

	ECG	CKG	Lactate production
Induction (n=23)	6	19	6
Before surgery (n=20)	5	18	1
Post incision (n=45)	19	37	6

Using any of the ischemic markers as goal standard, we analyzed the simultaneous recordings of PCWP/CVP and stroke volume. Patients with normal PCWP
wave form demonstrated an even distribution of values with changes from awake
between -14 and +21 mm Hg. The distribution of ischemic and non-ischemic events
were similar. Thus, an increase in PCWP by 8 mm Hg or more was associated with
a 43% likelihood of ischemia. In comparison, a reduction of PCWP by 1 mm Hg or
more, predicted ischemia in 54% of observations.

Thirteen percent of all observations were associated with abnormal PCWP
wave form. In these instances, the PCWP had a high predicitive value. Thus, 15
of 17 episodes (88%) with a rise in PCWP of 8 mm Hg or more and appearance of
abnormal wave form were associated with ischemia.

With onset of ischemia, CVP correlated closely with PCWP (CVP = 0.3xPCWP+
+ 1.9, r=0.853). As seen from the regression line equation, the incremental
rise in CVP was however 3/10 of the rise in PCWP, indicating a resolution which
is too low also in the presence of abnormal wave form. The change in stroke
volume measured during ischemia did not differ from the mean value obtained

during the non-ischemic periods.

In summary, the PCWP was a good indicator of ischemia, provided its rise was associated with appearance of abnormal wave form. Otherwise, its predictability was comparable to throwing a dice. CVP or stroke volume did not provide any additional value for the detection of ischemia.

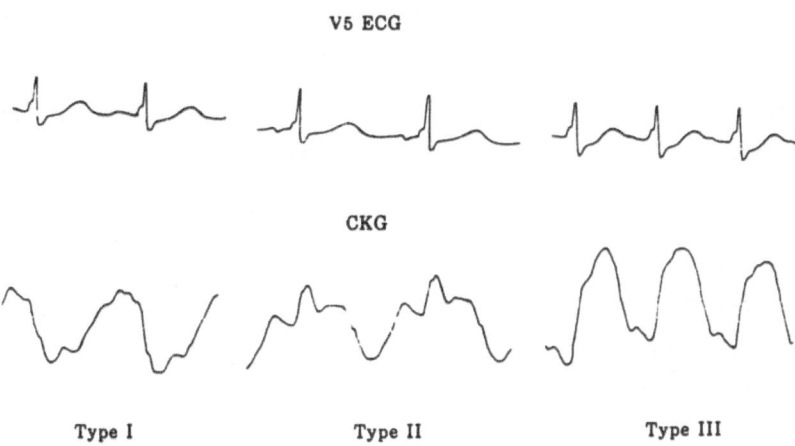

Fig 4. Development of partial (type II) and total systolic outward motion (type III) as detected by the CKG. ECG abnormality did not develop until total outward motion was recorded.

REFERENCES

1. Slogoff, S. and Keats, A.S.: Anesthesiology 62: 107-114, 1985.
2. Boucher, C.A., Brewster, D.C., Darling, R.C., et al: N. Engl. J. Med. 312: 389-394, 1985.
3. Hertzer,N.R., Beven, E.G., Young, J.R., et al: Ann. Surg. 199: 223-233.
4. Hertzer,N.R.: Surgery 93: 97-101.
5. Forrester, J.S., Wyatt, H.L., Tyberg, J.V., et al: Circulation 54: 64-70, 1976.
6. Picano, E., Morales, M-A., Distante, A., et al: Am. Heart J. 111: 688-691, 1986.
7. Kotrly, K.J., Kotter, G.S., Mortara, D. and Kampine, J.P.: Anesth. Analg. 63: 343-345.
8. Bellows, W.H., Bode, R.H., Levy, J.H., et al: Anesthesiology 60: 155-158, 1984.
9. Matsuma, M, Osa, Y., Strom, J., et al: Am. J. Cardiol. 46: 95-105, 1980.
10. Kaplan, J.A. and King, S.B.: Anesthesiology 45:570-574, 1976.
11. Silverberg, R.A., Diamond, G.A., Vas, R., et al: Criculation 61: 579-589, 1980.
12. Burke, J.F., Morganroth, J., Soffer, J., et al: Am. Heart J. 107: 718-725, 1984.
13. Weiner, A.W.: JACC 6: 502-509, 1985.
14. Coriat, P., Harari, M., Daloz, M., Viars, P.: Acta Anaestheiol. Scand. 26: 287-290, 1982.

EFFECT OF INHALATIONAL ANESTHETICS ON CARDIAC CONDUCTION

J. ZAIDAN

From clinical experience we know that inhalational anesthetics change heart rate and rhythm. Investigations concerning these changes study three different levels of effects of anesthetics on cardiac conduction. One type of investigation studies the effects of anesthetic agents in a single type of heart cell, the second type looks at the isolated heart preparation, and the third type observes the intact animal. All three types of studies are necessary in order to understand how changes in cardiac rate and rhythm occur in our anesthetized patients.

Many of the studies of cardiac conduction are performed with His-bundle recordings. These studies require specialized equipment and cannot be used for clinical care, but they answer many questions posed by the clinician. Atlee, et al, studied halothane anesthetized dogs and found that halothane increased the time for an impulse to be conduced from the SA node to the Bundle of His (the AH interval).(1) This interval further increased in the presence of rapid atrial pacing. Similar to the findings with the AH interval, the HV interval (the time for an impulse to traverse the Bundle of His and the purkinje fibers) also increased. The HV interval, while it did not further lengthen with rapid atrial pacing, increased with the administration of propranolol. Atropine did not change the effect of halothane on the HV interval, indicating that the effect is not parasympathetically mediated. Morrow, et al, anesthetized dogs with pentobarbital, 20-30 mg/kg, and found that halothane prolonged AH intervals before vagotomy, but not after vagotomy.(2) The authors concluded that halothane decreases heart rate by slowing AH conduction, and that this effect must have an intact Vagus nerve. The difference in the two studies could be secondary to the barbiturate. Turner, et al, found that halothane slowed conduction, and shortened ventricular functional refractory periods if the dogs did not

have basal barbiturate anesthesia.(3) Halothane given to dogs
administered intermittent barbiturates did not cause changes in
conduction and ventricular functional refractory periods. In an earlier
study involving barbiturates, Urthaler, et al, discovered that
pentobarbital, 30 mg/kg, administered to dogs had negative chronotropic
and dromotropic effects that transiently blocked the usual response to
vagal stimulation.(4) It is, therefore, obvious that the model in which
the investigation occurs affects the outcome. Enflurane reportedly
causes an increase in the AH interval without change in the HV interval
and isoflurane apparently has no effect on these intervals.(5,6) A
recent study by Atlee, et al, reveals that the inhalational anesthetic,
itself, does not the prolong conduction times.(7) Chronically
instrumented dogs were studied awake and then at 3 different MAC
levels. Enflurane and halothane increased conduction times at the
lowest MAC level and isoflurane increased conduction time at the highest
MAC level. Increasing the anesthetic depth with enflurane and halothane
did not further increase the conduction times. Interestingly,
administering beta and vagal blockade before anesthesia created the same
changes in AH and HV intervals as adding the anesthetic agents. Adding
anesthetic agents after beta and vagal blockade did not further change
the conduction times. In the intact animal, enflurane, isoflurane and
halothane appear to have secondary effects on cardiac conduction system
that act through the sympathetic and parasympathetic systems.

    Halothane has effects on conduction also at the cellular level. In
two separate studies, Hauswirth found differential effects of halothane
within the heart.(8,9) The SA node develops a dose dependent decrease
in the slope of phase four depolarization. Maximal diastolic potential
approaches the threshold potential, and action potential overshoot
decreases. Surprisingly, halothane has little effect on atrial
fibers. Halothane causes the resting membrane potential of purkinje
fibers to become more negative in a dose dependent manner. Purkinje
fiber action potential duration decreases in the presence of
halothane. Ventricular fibers had no change in resting membrane
potential, but halothane caused a decrease in the action potential
overshoot and in the action potential duration. In a more recent study,
Bosnjak, et al, investigated the effects of halothane, enflurane, and
isoflurane on SA nodal cells.(10) All of these agents decrease heart

172

rate, the slope of phases 4 and 0 of depolarization, and action
potential duration. These effects were dose related.

It is exceedingly difficult to determine the effect of these agents
in the human, because almost all of these studies have been performed in
dogs and guinea pigs. If an unpremedicated patient receives halothane,
this patient most likely will have slowing of the heart rate, nodal
dysrhythmias, and probably a high likelihood of ventricular escape
beats, especially if the patient is not well ventilated. Enflurane
could be associated with approximately stable heart rates, and a
likelihood of atrial dysrhythmias. Isoflurane in non-beta-blocked
patients is associated with increases in heart rate and stable
conduction if the increased heart rate does not cause a detrimental
change in the myocardial oxygen supply demand ratio.

REFERENCES

1. Atlee, J.L., Rusy, B.F. Anesthesiology 36: 112-118, 1972.
2. Morrow, D.H., Logic J.R., Haley, J.V. Anesth Analg 56:187-193,
    1977.
3. Turner, L.A., Zuperku, E.J., Purtock, R.V. Kampine, J.P. Anesth
    Analg 59:327-334, 1980.
4. Urthale, F., Krames, B.L. James, T.N. Cardiovasc Res 8:46-57, 1974.
5. Atlee, J.L., Rusy, B.F. Anesthesiology 47:498. 1977.
6. Blitt, C.D., Raessler, K.L., Wightman, M.A., et al. Anesthesiology
    50:210-212, 1979.
7. Atlee, J.L., Brownlee, S.W., Burstrom, R.E. Anesthesiology 64:703-
    710, 1986.
8. Hauswirth, O, Schaer, H: J Pharmacol Exper Ther 158:36-39, 1967.
9. Hauswirth, O. Circulation Res 24:745-750, 1969.
10. Bosnjak, Z.J., Kampine, J.P. Anesthesiology 58:314-321, 1983.

ISOFLURANE AND CORONARY BLOOD FLOW REGULATION

Sebastian Reiz, MD, PhD

A large body of animal experimentation demonstrates that isoflurane is a coronary vasodilator with a potency considerably greater than halothane or enflurane. In comparison with adenosine and dipyridamole, isoflurane is however, a weak coronary dilator (1,2).

In patients with coronary artery disease subjected to peripheral arterial surgery or coronary artery revascularization, Reiz and coworkers (3) and Moffitt and colleagues (4) respectively, found isoflurane to decrease coronary perfusion pressure without altering coronary blood flow. In both studies, myocardial oxygen extraction fell profoundly, indicating a direct action of the anesthetic upon coronary vascular tone and auto-regulation (Table 1). These changes occurred regardless of the use of betablocking agents, differences in premedication and induction agents or the presence of nitrous oxide. In addition, a significant number of patients were found to be ischemic as diagnosed by lactate balance studies and/or electrocardiographic changes. In the study by Reiz et al, ischemia persisted in some patients despite normalization of coronary perfusion pressure, suggesting redistribution of coronary blood flow as one contributing mechanism for the development of ischemia.

Table 1. Percentage change in coronary hemodynamics and myocardial oxygenation induced by isoflurane in patients with coronary artery disease.

	MAP	CBF	$M\dot{V}O_2$	CSO_2 cont	Ischemia
Reiz et al (1983)	-40*	-7	-36*	+48*	10/21
Moffitt et al (1986)	-33*	-12	-43*	+56*	3/10

MAP-mean arterial pressure, CBF-coronary blood flow, $M\dot{V}O_2$-myocardial oxygen consumption, CSO_2 cont-coronary sinus oxygen content. *-significant changes from awake.

In a recently completed randomized, double blind study, Reiz and coworkers compared the systemic and coronary hemodynamic effects of halothane and isoflurane. The anesthetic agents were administered in nitrous oxide/oxygen (60/40) after induction with fentanyl/thiopentone to morphine premedicated patients with coronary artery disease subjected to peripheral arterial revascularization. Coronary perfusion pressure was controlled with phenylephrine and pulmonary capillary wedge pressure with nitroglycerine, if indicated by hypotension or cardiac failure. Eighteen of the nineteen patients needed phenylephrine before incision to maintain a blood pressure above 70% of the awake value. Hemodynamics were significantly more abnormal in halothane patients despite a higher dose of vasopressor. Despite the use of multiple induction drugs and vasopressor therapy, the coronary hemodynamic effects of the anesthetic agents were comparable to those previously reported in individuals with coronary artery disease (3-6). Thus, halothane produced a decline in coronary blood flow parallelling the reduction in perfusion pressure. In comparison, coronary blood flow remained unchanged and myocardial oxygen extraction decreased significantly after isoflurane, indicating coronary vasodilation (Table 2).

Table 2. Percentage change in coronary hemodynamics following halothane and isoflurane in patients with coronary artery disease.

	DAP	PCWP	CBF	$M\dot{V}O_2$	MO_2 extr
Halothane (n=10)	-18*	+65*	-32*	-40*	-8
Isoflurane (n=9)	-5	+20*	-1	-18*	-15*

DAP-diastolic arterial pressure, PCWP-pulmonary capillary wedge pressure, CBF-coronary blood flow, $M\dot{V}O_2$-myocardial oxygen consumption, MO_2 extr-myocardial oxygen extraction. *-significantly changed from awake values.

Two other clinical studies of isoflurane, carried out by the group headed by Tarnow, obtained data compatible with the above studies, though they were interpreted by the authors to be in conflict. Hess and coworkers (7) studied the effects of adding isoflurane or halothane to patients in whom surgical stimulation during flunitrazepam-fentanyl anesthesia produced hypertension. Ischemia, as detected by the electrocardiogram, was present in 3 of 20 patients, two of whom received isoflurane, the remaining received halothane. The ECG changes disappeared with increasing depth of anesthesia, reducing mean arterial pressure. In this situation, the reduction in myocardial oxygen demand produced by isoflurane clearly must have outweighed any adverse redistributive effect of the anesthetic agent. It does not, however, argue against impairment of coronary autoregulation.

In the second study (8), Tarnow and colleagues investigated the effects of atrial pacing on the V5 ST segment before and during isoflurane-nitrous oxide-oxygen anesthesia in patients scheduled for coronary artery revascularization. They found patients to have significantly less ST depression when paced to the same heart rate during anesthesia as when awake. Also coronary perfusion pressure, filling pressure and rate pressure product (RPP), and thus myocardial oxygen demand were significantly lower than during the conscious state.

Tarnow presented ECG data from 13 patients. In nine patients, the decreases of RPP and ST segment correlated closely. In three patients, the ST segment abnormality was unchanged despite reduction in RPP and in the last patient, the ST segment depression increased (Fig. 1). Thus, four patients did not demonstrate improvement in their index of myocardial ischemia despite a reduction in their index of myocardial oxygen demand. In these patients, it is not possible to exclude the role of coronary redistribution as a contributing factor for ischemia.

Fig 1. Rate-prssure product plotted versus changes in ST segment of the V5 ECG in patients with coronary artery disease and during isoflurane anesthesia. Angina threshold was determined by atrial pacing awake. The heart was paced to the same heart rate during anesthesia. Four patients did not improve their index of myocardial ischemia despite a reduction in myocardial oxygen demand. Data re-plotted from Tarnow et al (8).

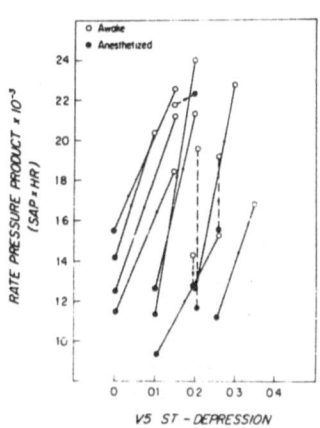

Confirmatory evidence of the role of redistribution of coronary blood flow during isoflurane anesthesia has recently been obtained in animal models. Buffington and coworkers (9) performed acute experiments in dogs three or four weeks after ameroid induced occlusion of the left anterior descending coronary artery (LAD) which permits collateralization of the LAD territory. They demonstrated that isoflurane produced redistribution of blood flow from the subendocardium of the collateral dependent zone to the epicardium of normal myocardium. In addition abnormal wall motion appeared in the collateralized area, suggesting ischemia.

Priebe conducted cross-over experiments with halothane and isoflurane in dogs with acutely constricted LAD coronary arteries. At comparable perfusion pressure, heart rate and left ventricular end-diastolic pressure, coronary blood flow to the area supplied by the stenosed artery was higher and shortening was greater during halothane than during isoflurane. In contrast, flow to the area supplied by the non-stenosed circumflex artery was higher during isoflurane anesthesia. Regional function in this area remained normal.

In summary, isoflurane, similar to other coronary vasodilators (10-13), can cause maldistribution of blood flow, despite lowering myocardial oxygen demand. Patients with a collateralized area, particularly if this is perfused from a stenotic artery, may be at greatest risk of developing ischemia in the colleteralized zone. It is also likely, that a stenosis becomes pressure dependent at a relatively higher blood pressure, lower heart rate and/or lower left ventricular filling pressure if such a patient is anesthetized with a coronary vasodilating agent than with one that does not interfere with coronary autoregulation. Since the anatomy of most patients with coronary artery disease subjected to non-cardiac surgery is not known, it appears prudent to maintain heart rate, blood pressure and filling pressure close to their normal values if isoflurane is selected as the anesthetic agent.

REFERENCES
1. Tarnow, J., Eberlein, H.J. and Oser, G. et al. Anaesthetist 26: 220-230, 1977.
2. Sybert, P.E., Hickey, R.F. and Hoar, P.F. et al. Anesthesiology 59, A24 (abstr), 1983.
3. Reiz, S., Bålfors, E., Sörensen, M.B. and Ariola Jr, S. et al. Anesthesiology 59: 91-97, 1983.
4. Moffitt, E.A., Barker, R.A. and Glenn, J.J. et al. Anesth. Analg. 65: 53-61, 1986.
5. Wilkinson, P.L., Hamilton, W.K. and Moyers, J.R. et al. J. Thorac. Cardiovasc. Surg. 82: 372, 1981.
6. Reiz, S., Bålfors, E. and Gustavsson, B. et al. Acta Anaesth. Scand. 26: 133-138, 1982.
7. Hess, W., Arnold, B. and Schulte-Sasse, U. et al. Anesth. Analg. 62: 15-20, 1983.

8. Tarnow, J., Markschies-Hornung, A. and Schulte-Sasse, U. Anesthesiology 64: 147-156, 1986.
9. Buffington, C.W., Romson, J.L. and Duttlinger, N.C. Anesthesiology 63, A9 (abstr), 1985.
10. Becker, L.C. J. Clin. Invest. 58: 1287-1296, 1976.
11. Becker, L.C. Circulation 57: 1103-1110, 1978.
12. Henry, P.D., Shuchleib, R. and Borda, L.J. et al. Circ. Res. 43: 372-380, 1978.
13. Chiariello, M., Gold, H.K. and Leinbach, R.C. et al. Circulation 54: 766-773, 1976.

WILDLIFE CAPTURE: ARE THE STRESSES APPLICABLE TO HUMANS?

J.C. HAIGH

INTRODUCTION
     The capture of wildlife, whether in zoos or in free ranging situations, involves either the physical or chemical restraint of animals. Either method places stresses upon the animal which may lead to the condition known as capture myopathy (CM). This condition has many characteristics associated with malignant hyperthermia (MH) of humans as well as porcine stress syndrome (or MH) of pigs and white muscle disease of cattle. In some phase of all of these conditions pathological myodegenerative changes occur. The condition in man to which CM may be most closely related is so-called march myoglobinuria or exertional rhabdomyolosis seen in untrained athletes or military recruits, especially at high ambient temperatures (1,2).

     Capture myopathy is also known by a variety of other names which include overstraining disease, stress myopathy, transport myopathy, white muscle disease, post-capture myopathy, exertional rhabdomyolosis, vangspier sindroom, overstraining syndrome and leg paralysis.

     Capture myopathy has been recognized in many species of animal from around the world (3). Among mammals virtually all of these species are herbivorous and many are also prey species. There are no clearly demonstrated cases of CM in carnivores. CM has also been reported in several species of bird.

PREDISPOSING FACTORS
     The manifestations of CM vary according to several factors. These include the species, the method of capture, the season and ambient temperature, and both the mental state and physical condition of the animal. No doubt there are individual variations in susceptibility.

Species

Some species of animal are notoriously more nervous and therefore more likely to succumb to this condition than others. Pronghorn antelope, among north american species are particularly prone. Black bears, which have been captured for years in several different stressful ways, have never been reported to have had CM. The degree of physical fitness and acclimatization are important components in the development of CM. The grazing or browsing herbivore has no need to keep fit in the athletic sense whereas the carnivore, whether lion or wolf must be capable of tremendous athletic achievement in order to earn its meals. It may be that different species of animal have different muscle types which may effect their susceptibility. Other than in pigs there are no reports of individual variability, but the possibility exists.

During extensive studies on the physiology of CM Harthoorn found that physically conditioned wildebeest, eland and zebra showed a decreasing incidence of CM as they remained in captivity and went through training periods. Certainly the parallel condition in horses known as paralytic myoglobinuria, which occurs in rested horses, subjected to sudden exercise, but not in those in training, lends credence to the notion that the athletically fit animal is less likely to develop the condition.

The method of restraint plays an important role in the outcome of any wildlife capture routine. The two main methods are of course physical restraint and chemical immobilization, which may often be combined. CM has been documented in both and the use of drugs probably does not increase the incidence of CM. Rather it is the choice of an inappropriate method for the given species in a given set of environmental conditions which is likely to lead to trouble.

The length and severity of chases will effect their outcome, as will the degree of acclimatization of the animal and the type of actual capture method used. Research into the effects of various types of chase have shown that short (2 km) chases at high speed caused a very marked drop in blood ph to levels below 7.0. The ph was not as low after slower, longer chases, but there were other detrimental effects which included myoglobinemia and hemoglobinemia (1). There is a marked rise in the incidence of CM in moose immobilized from a helicopter if the chase lasts longer than 2 min. (Haigh, unpubl.).

CM has been seen in instances where no chase at all was involved. The capture of bighorn sheep (Ovis canadensis) by drop nets has led to CM (4). Similarly the condition has been seen in snow geese captured under cannon nets (5). In these and other similar cases it is likely that isometric muscle contraction played a role in development of the condition. Severe isometric exercise in human patients dosed with phenyclidine and restrained with ropes, has been reported to lead to markedly elevated levels of muscle enzymes (6).

Fear

An important trigger for CM is fear or terror. These, acknowledged at first by visual and auditory receptors will activate the sympathico-adrenal system and through the actions of both epinephrine and norepinephrine have effects upon blood pressure, blood flow to various organs, and carbo-hydrate metabolism. The secretion of glucocorticoids from the adrenal cortex, also stimulated by fear, has immediate effects upon carbohydrate metabolism.

Temperature

The environmental temperature also plays a key role in the development of CM. If captures are carried out at high temperature, CM is much more likely to develop. Equally important is what may be termed the net temperature, which is a combination of the environmental temperature and the animal's ability to cool itself. If a heavy winter coat insulates an animal on a relatively warm day evaporative cooling may be minimal. The use of drugs that depress respiration will suppress cooling via the respiratory tree. Improper crating of animals being transported can also precipitate CM by preventing cooling.

Nutrition

The nutritional status of the animals is also important in terms of resistance to CM. Not only is the general physical condition important but the intake of both selenium and vitamin E and their availability in forage play a role. Both are antioxidants and are important in the protecti of cell membranes. Selenium is incorporated in glutathione peroxidase molecules which play an integral part in the reduction of organic hydro-peroxides and hydrogen peroxide which may build up during exercise (7) (Fig 1). Levels of 85 i.u. of vitamin E per kg of feed have been shown to protect white-tailed deer from CM (8) and tissue selenium levels are

inversely correlated with the incidence of CM in African capture exercises
(1). Generous levels of vitamin E in feed have been shown to protect
against CM even if selenium levels are low (8).

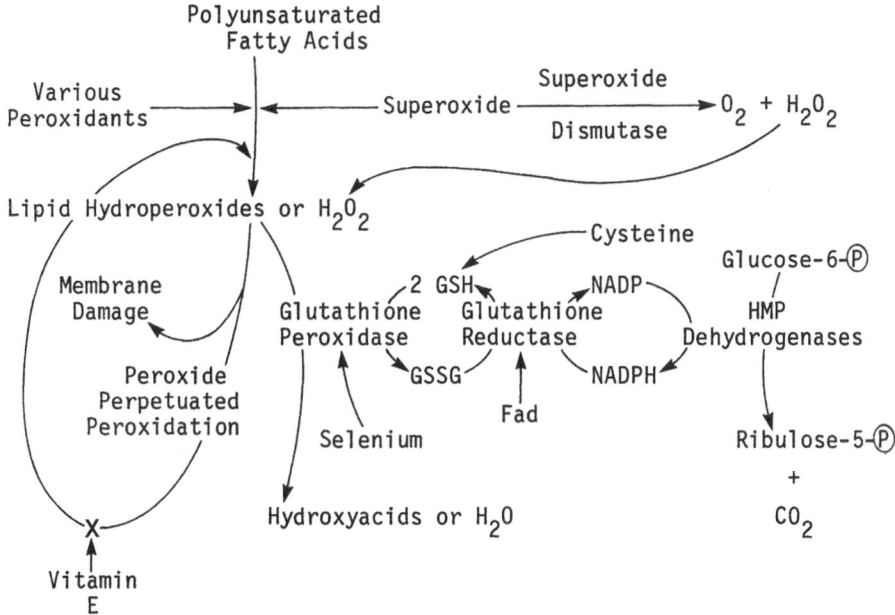

Fig. 1. The erythrocyte glutathione peroxidase system. (Reprinted with
permission from ref. 9).

The final disposition of the animal will govern its recovery. There
was a 4.2% CM related mortality among pronghorn antelope captured and
released whereas the same method of capture followed by transport led to
a 23% CM related mortality (10).

A good example of the effect of different capture methods on the outcome in a single species is shown by the caribou which has been
successfully captured by a variety of different methods. These have
included the use of ropes from boats at river and lake crossings, the
use of nets across established trails at the edge of frozen lakes, net
guns fired from helicopters and drug immobilization of caribou moved slowly
toward a hidden marksman (11). A high incidence of CM was reported after
caribou had been chased by helicopter and darted after prolonged chases.
When immobilized animals struggled under the influence of inadequate drug
doses the incidence of CM rose (12).

Immobilizing Drugs

There is no evidence to suggest that any of the centrally acting drugs use in wildlife immobilization have any direct effect upon the incidence of CM. Indeed in many species their use has eliminated the fear responses evident when animals are captured by physical means alone. The extra-pyramidal effects, especially disruption of thermo-regulation, produced by the phenothiazines may be important in the ultimate survival of the subject. The use of phenothiazines should be avoided at extremes of temperature. The butyrophenone related neurologic malignant syndrome in man (13) has no reported parallel in animals.

Perhaps the most commonly used of all the immobilizing narcotics is etorphine hydrochloride. This drug causes tachycardia and increased blood pressure which is particularly pronounced in equidae (14). Underdosing with narcotics is widely recognized as a cause of overexcitement that can lead to hyperthermia and overexertion (15). The respiratory depressant effects of the potent narcotics etorphine, fentanyl and carfentanyl are not very pronounced at doses needed for immobilization - at least not in herbivores. The use of the butyrophenone azaperone has been shown in some species to counteract the depressant effects of the narcotics through its α receptor blockade, thus decreasing the trigger level raised by the narcotic (15). Xylazine hydrochloride is a central α2 andrenergic agonist and causes reduced blood pressure and bradycardia when used alone. This drug is very popular when used as a synergist with either narcotics or cyclohexamines and the cardiovascular effects are not usually seen if the drug is used in this fashion (15). Recent interest in still investigational serotonin antagonists may further enhance the use of narcotics by reducing the immobilizing dose by as much as 70% (16).

Studies of the effects of cyclohexamines in conjunction with sedatives on pH and acid base balance have been carried out in captive bears and lions. The effects were minimal (17, 18).

AETIOLOGY AND PATHOPHYSIOLOGY

As with many disease conditions there is no simple single cause of capture myopathy. Rather it is a medusa headed complex of factors which may act in concert or singly to variously effect the outcome. In humans and pigs the triggering mechanisms of genetially determined malignant hyper-thermia have been described as potent volatile anesthetics, succinylcholine,

decamethonium, environmental stress and excitement (1,2). Fear and/or
vigorous exercise are the two most common stimulants associated with the
development of CM. They have effects on the cardiovascular system, heat
dissipation, and the muscle pump.

Cardio-vascular Function

Detailed studies of the effects of capture on a full range of cardiovascular functions have only been made on a limited number of animals. All
of these were carried out by Harthoorn (1).

He studied cardiac function in eland wildebeest and zebra that had
been physically restrained. The effects included a marked fall in cardiac
output over the first half hour after capture. In general levels fell from
about 10 to 13 1/min immediately after capture to 5 1/min or less. There
was a simultaneous development of pulmonary hypertension and systemic hypotension. The pulmonary hypertension was not always evident just after capture,
but within 30 to 60 min it had risen to levels as high as 100 mm Hg.

Several different observations of the effect of capture and adrenaline
induced stress on immobilized animals upon electro-cardiogram were noted.
These included inverted T waves associated with cardiac ischemia in eland,
sino-auricular and atrio-ventricular block, ectopic arrhthymias, paroxysmal
tachycardia, blending of RS and T waves associated with hyperkalemia and
hypocalcemic effects of slurring of the QRS complex with prolongation of the
QT interval (1).

The effects of physical and chemical restraint upon acid base balance and
lactate levels were also studied by Harthoorn (1) and have been investigated
in moose (Haigh unpubl.) The basic change was a metabolic acidosis. In
the most severe cases in zebra, associated with short intense chases pH
values fell below 7.0 and in some animals as low as 6.50. In some zebras
pH fell further in the 30 min after capture. In moose immobilized from a
helicopter with fentanyl and xylazine there was also a metabolic acidosis.
pH levels did not fall below 7.033 (Haigh unpubl.).

Hyperthermia

Hyperthermia is one of the most important problems associated with wild
animal capture. Not only is it seen when ambient temperature is high, but
it can also occur on cold days when internally generated heat is improperly
dissipated. This may be due not only to reduced tissue perfusion but also
to the insulating effects of heavy winter coats on relatively warm days.
Heat production due to muscle activity and the absorption of ambient heat

raise the muscle temperature and speed up local chemical reactions. If the cardio-vascular system is functioning properly this heat is rapidly removed from the muscle. The effects of capture on the cardiovascular system mitigate against efficient heat removal. Some of the drugs used for chemical immobilization are also known to adversely effect thermo-regulation.

The Muscle Pump

The muscle pump functions during exercise. During the relaxation phase blood flows into muscle, but it is squeezed out during contraction and even arterial blood cannot enter the muscles (2).

In the normal resting body there is about 15% of total blood volume in the muscle mass. Just after exercise this can rise to 25%. During the chase phase of capture the muscle pump is still working, but in the frightene animal, or one undergoing isotonic contraction, the pump is lost and the reduced tissue perfusion leads to decreased heat dissipation and local hypoxia, which in turn leads to lowered pH. Conversley in the chemically immobilized animal the muscles may be fully relaxed and an increased blood flow to them may occur with no return pump action. Because of reduced blood pressure and increased pooling there is decreased heat dissipation and hypoxia leading to the same end result (Fig. 2) (2).

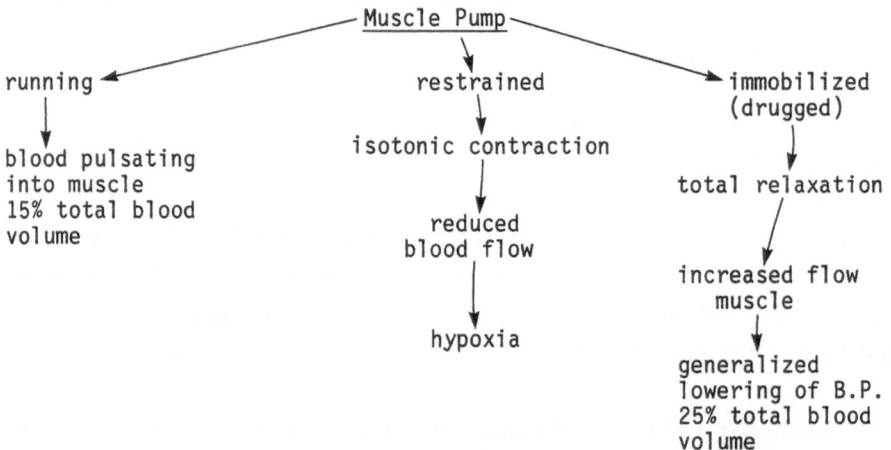

Fig. 2. Flow-chart for general concept of action and problems that develop with regard to the muscle pump. (Reprinted with permission from ref. 2).

MANIFESTATIONS OF CAPTURE MYOPATHY

Most authors agree that CM can be broadly divided into four different manifestations. In general the subdivisions suggested by Harthoorn (1) of per-acute, acute, subacute and chronic forms cover the range. A series of descriptive names developed by Spraker (2) also has useful aspects. The latter system divides CM into 4 syndromes. These are Peracute Death, Acute Death, Ataxic Myoglobinuric, and Ruptured Muscle syndromes.

Peracute Capture Myopathy

In the peracute form the cause of death is ventricular fibrillation brought on by severe metabolic acidosis and concurrent hyperkalemia. Harthoorn has measured blood pH values in chased zebra as low as 6.50 (1). He also measured pO_2 and pCO_2 and found that during thermal panting soon after capture pCO_2 levels were elevated. The combination of metabolic and respiratory acidosis accounts for the hyperkalemia. This type of syndrome has been seen not only in freshly caught animals that died within a few hours of capture but also in animals that have recently been captured, appear to be in good condition, but suddenly fall and die when excited or re-stressed. In the latter case it has been suggested that a fresh surge of epinephrine and norepinephrine from the adrenal medulla has caused fibrillation in cardiac cells already sensitized by hyperkalemia (2).

Acute Capture Myopathy

In the acute form of CM a combination of severe metabolic acidosis, hyperthermia, acute adrenal exhaustion, shock and rhabdomyolosis are probably involved. Death occurs within a few hours of capture. Clinical manifestations of this form include depression, shallow rapid breathing, tachycardia, oliguria, muscular stiffness, usually elevated body temperature, and often pulmonary edema (1,2,3).

The depressed blood pH values associated with metabolic acidosis may not be as low as those measured in muscle tissue itself (1). Local ischemia and anoxia will further exacerbate the situation and cause local production of lactic acid, membrane damage, fibre rupture, potassium and myoglobin release. Elevated serum lactic levels will in turn lead to intravascular hemolysis.

In tropical conditions, where dietary potassium may be deficient, adequate vasodilation may not occur in the absence of this ion (19).

186

On post-mortem examination the most common lesions include pulmonary edema and severe congestion of the small intestine and liver (2). Some degree of rhabdomyolisis will also be found.

Sub-acute Capture Myopathy

The sub-acute or ataxic-myoglobinuric syndrome is associated with the results of muscle and organ damage (1). The clinical signs may range from mild to very severe and animals may survive for several days but die despite treatment. The clinical signs include lameness, torticollis, inability to rise and myoglobinuria. Analysis of blood enzymes reveals damage to skeletal muscle and major organs. In particular serum glutamic oxalacetic transaminase, creatin pyrokinase, lactic dehydrogenase and blood urea nitrogen and creatinine levels are elevated.

A decrease in renal blood flow caused by both epinephrine and norepinephrine can lead via tubular necrosis to a failing kidney. This situation is exacerbated by the deposition of both hemoglobin and myoglobin in the glomeruli and in time myoglobinuria becomes evident.

Post-mortem examination usually reveals both kidney and widespread muscle damage (1,2,3). The muscle lesions are usually bilateral, but not necessarily symmetrical. The muscle damage may be so severe that massive muscle rupture occurs. This is often, but not always, seen in the gastro-cnemius muscles (Fig 3 a,b). Spraker (2) has separated this syndrome from other manifestations of CM.

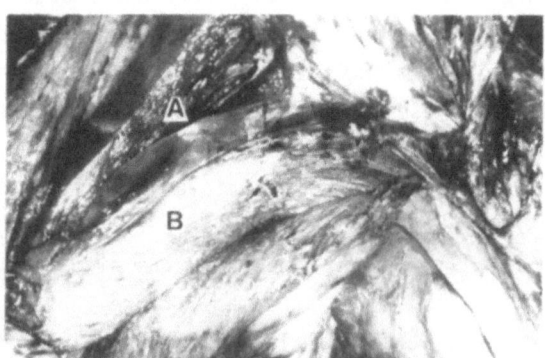

Fig. 3a. a) Gross post mortem appearance of adjacent normal looking (A) and pale white (B) muscles in the hind leg of an elk that died 3 days after going down with CM.

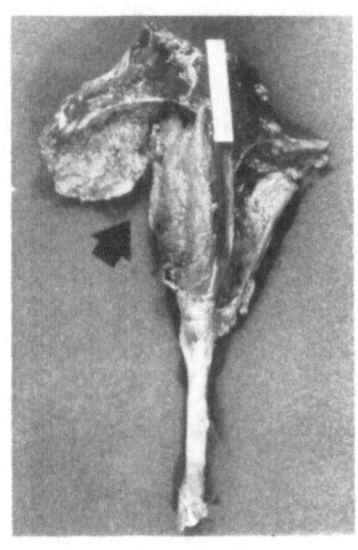

Fig. 3b. Ruptured gastrocnemius muscle (arrow) of a white-tailed deer that died of CM (Photo courtesy G. Wobeser).

Chronic Capture Myopathy

The chronic or indefinite form of CM is considered to be associated with myocardial damage and has not been clearly demonstrated. It may be characterized by sudden death, following renewed stress of animals that have survived the initial capture for several weeks or even months. Post-mortem examination shows fibrosed heart lesions (1,3).

TREATMENT AND PREVENTION

Prevention is usually considered the best form of treatment. In effected animals a considerable variety of treatments have been tried. Their success is dependent both upon the type of CM that is being treated and the extent to which they can be administered without further exacerbating the condition.

The most dramatic reports of treatment have involved the use of 4-6 mEq/kg of Na bicarbonate solution intravenously to animals with profound acidemia. In a controlled test on zebra that had been subjected to chase and exhibited blood pH values below 6.87 3 untreated animals died and all 6 of the treated animals recovered (1). Others using various formulations of bicarbonate have also had success (20,21).

In controlled trials on chemically immobilized helicopter chased moose the use of Na bicarbonate solution at 4-6 mEq/kg was tested. All the moose had pretreatment arterial pH values above 7.032. There was no statistical difference between pH values in treated or untreated moose 30 min after infusion. All values rose toward normal during this time and this probably reflects the fact the animals were able to compensate for their acidosis when pH values did not fall too far (Haigh unpubl).

The use of vitamin E/Selenium injections may well be mandatory in animals captured in areas where these dietary components are deficient. In cattle with white muscle disease its use is standard, and prophylactic injections of vitamin E/Selenium preparations are routinely used in some zoos to prevent this syndrome in juvenile ungulates (21,22). Other drugs that have been tried with greater or lesser success have included vitamin B12, calcium boroglucinate, corticosteroids, detoxicants, and antihistamines (3). Recently the use of fluxinin meglumine was reported to have helped in a clinical case (in conjunction with other treatments) (23).

Dantrolene sodium is well recognized as a crucial component of malignant hyperthermia treatment in man (24). This drug is also used prophylactically via the oral route in swine and horses (25,26). The administration of commercially available dantrolene by injection to free ranging wildlife would not only be awkward, but also prohibitively expensive. The extraction of the active component from the oral preparation has recently been reported (27). I have tried this preparation on a few occasions in zoo animals that seemed to be at risk of developing CM, but there are no data to support any conclusions other than the fact that the animals lived, which they might have done anyway. If animals are being baited under drop nets prior to capture it would certainly be feasible to prophylactically administer dantrolene in the feed.

The most important method of dealing with CM is to prevent it. One of the simplest methods of prevention is to employ the T, T and T method described by Harthoorn (1,28). Essentially this method involves the enticement of animals into large corrals followed by their gradual taming and their handling without hurry. The 3 T's stand for training, taming and tempo. Similar techniques can readily be used for many species. In almost any climate there are times of year when feed is at a premium and animals will enter corrals. The use of anxyolitics such as Haloperidol has been described (20) and can add to the success of the operation. If these methods cannot be employed the choice of the correct method, at the right time of day, in the appropriate season of the year must be made.

Perseus, who made himself invisible and slew Medusa by looking at her indirectly and cutting off her head, escaped by climbing on the winged horse Pegasus who emerged from the stump. A parallel approach to wild animals using subtlety may go a long way to preventing disaster.

CONCLUSION

Although there exist many similarities between malignant hyperthermia and capture myopathy these seem to reflect the limited ways in which the cardiovascular system and the muscles can react to adverse stimuli. The underlying physiological end results, especially in striated muscle, are no doubt almost identical, but the triggering mechanisms are somewhat different. In MH a failure of the Calcium pump in the sarcoplasmic reticulum is the physiological event that fails (24). A complex series of adverse steps are involved in the development of CM. The prevention of CM by training cannot be applied to the human patient in whom malignant hyperthermia is a genetically determined condition. On the other hand march myoglobinuria may well be a mild form of CM.

REFERENCES

1. Harthoorn, A.M., Quinquennial Report, Transvaal Nature Conservation Division, 1976.
2. Spraker, T.R. In: Chemical Immobilization of North American Wildlife (Eds. L. Nielsen, J.C. Haigh and M.E. Fowler), The Wisconsin Humane Society, 1982, pp. 83-118.
3. Chalmers, G.A. and Barrett, M.W. In: Noninfectious Diseases of Wildlife (Eds. G.L. Hoff and J.W. Davis), Iowa State University Press, 1982, pp. 84-94.
4. Spraker, T.R. In: Pathology of Skeletal Muscle of Animals. 26th Ann. Seminar Amer. Coll of Vet. Pathologists, 1975.
5. Wobeser, G.A. Diseases of Wild Waterfowl. Plenum Publishing corp., New York, N.Y., 1981.
6. Aronow, R. and Done, A.K. J. Amer. Coll. Emergency Physicians, 7: 56-59, 1978.
7. Brady, P.S., Brady, L., Whetter, P.A., Ullrey, D.A. and Fay, L.D. Nutr. 108: 1439-1448, 1978.
8. Ullrey, D.E., Schmitt, S.M., Cooley, T.A., Ku, P.K. and Whetter, P.A. In: Proceedings Amer. Assoc. Zoo Vets, 1984, pp. 37-39.
9. Brady, P.S., Shelle, J.E. and Ullrey, D.E. Am. J. Vet. Res. 38: 1045-1047, 1977.
10. Chalmers, G.A. and Barrett, M.W. J. Amer. Vet. Med. Assoc. 171: 918-923, 1977.

190

11. Haigh, J.C. In: Proceedings Amer. Assoc. Zoo Vets, 1978, pp. 110-115.
12. Fuller, T. and Keith, L.B. J. Wildl. Manage. 45: 745-748, 1983.
13. Smego, R.A. and Durack, D.T. Arch. Intern. Med. 142: 1183-1185, 1982.
14. Daniel, M. and Ling, C.M. Vet. Rec. 90: 336-339, 1972.
15. Haigh, J.C. In: Chemical Immobilization of North American Wildlife (Eds L. Nielsen, J.C. Haigh and M.E. Fowler), The Wisconsin Humane Society, 1982, pp. 46-62.
16. Bailey, P.L., Port, J.D., Pace, N.L., Stanley, T.H. and Kimball, J. J. Wildl. Manage. 49: 931-934, 1985.
17. Bush, M., Custer, R.S. and Smith, E.E. J. Wildl. Dis. 16: 481-489, 1980.
18. Bush, M., Custer, R.S., Smeller, J.M., Bush, L.M., Seal, U.S., and Barton, R. J. Wildl. Dis. 14: 102-109, 1978.
19. Knochel, J.P. and Schlein, E.M. J. Clin. Investig. 51: 1750-1758, 1972.
20. Gericke, M.D., Hofmeyr, J.M. and Louw, G.N. Madoqua, 11: 5-18, 1978.
21. Blood, D.C., Radostits, O.M. and Henderson, J.A. Veterinary Medicine. Balliere Tindall. London 1983, pp. 1047-1054.
22. Klos, H.G. and Lang, E.M. Handbook of Zoo Medicine. Van Nostrand Reinhold Co., New York, 1976.
23. Kollias, G.V., Colahan, P.T. and Walsh, M.T. J. Amer. Vet. Med. Assoc. 183: 1334-1337, 1983.
24. Gregory, G.A. In: Anesthesia (Ed. R.D. Miller) 1981, pp. 1208-1212.
25. Harrison, G.G. Br. J. Anaesth. 49: 315, 1977.
26. Court, M.H., Engelking, L.R., Dodman, N.H. and Seeler, D.C. In: Proceedings, 2nd Intl. Cong. Vet. Anes. 1985, p. 103.
27. O'Brien, P.J. and Forsyth, G.W. Can. Vet. J. 24: 200, 1983.
28. Harthoorn, A.M. In: Chemical Immobilization of North American Game Animals. (Eds L. Nielsen, J.C. Haigh and M.E. Fowler), 1982, pp. 150-164.

NEONATAL ANESTHESIA

F. A. BERRY

The infant under one year of age presents a special challenge to
the anesthesiologist. There is no other time period where so many
changes occur so rapidly. This discussion will deal primarily with the
full term infant up to one year of age, but some mention will be made
of the premature infant. It will begin with the basic considerations
of an infant presenting for surgery and then proceed to a discussion of
the interaction of anesthetic agents and techniques with these basic
considerations. There are four basic considerations when an infant
presents with a surgical problem: (1) transition (fetal → newborn
state), (2) maturation (growth and development), (3) the surgical
defect and (4) associated congenital anomalies.

Transition refers to the changes that occur with the birth
process. The fetal state is one of dependency upon the placenta for
all functions. The newborn state is characterized by an abrupt loss of
this support organ and a rapid assumption of all body functions.
Transition has nothing to do with growth and development but comes
about through the enormous changes that occur in circulation and
ventilation. This discussion will center on three primary systems that
undergo transition: (1) the circulatory system, (2) the pulmonary
system, and (3) the renal system. The circulation abruptly changes at
birth from that of the fetus to the newborn because of alterations in
the three major shunts that are present within the circulation of the
fetus, i.e., placenta, foramen ovale, and ductus arteriosus. The fetus
has a relatively high pulmonary vascular resistance and a relatively
low systemic pressure. This leads to a higher pressure within the
right atrium than the left atrium, thereby shunting blood past the
right side of the circulation through the foramen ovale. The high

pulmonary vascular resistance also causes a shunting of blood from the right heart through the ductus arteriosus to the aorta. The amount of circulation to the lungs is approximately 10% of the output of the right heart. At birth there is an abrupt amputation of the placenta and a decrease in pulmonary vascular resistance as the lungs are expanded. In addition, there is an increase in systemic blood pressure. This results in the left atrial pressure exceeding the right atrial pressure and a functional closing of the foramen ovale. (Approximately 20% of adults have a probe patient foramen ovale). As the blood is oxygenated, the ductus arteriosus constricts and this leads to the mature circulation with no shunts. Varying degrees of hypoxia and acidosis can have an adverse effect upon the circulation in this period of transition. Acidosis and hypoxia cause an increase in pulmonary vascular resistance. This may result in a reopening of the ductus arteriosus and of the foramen ovale and a return to what has been termed "persistent pulmonary hypertension." There are basically two types of persistent pulmonary hypertension (also referred to as persistent fetal circulation): (1) a reactive pulmonary vascular bed, and (2) an absolute increase in the amount and distribution of the muscle content of the pulmonary vascular bed. A reactive pulmonary vascular bed may be found under circumstances such as asphyxia and meconium aspiration, as well as often being associated with the postoperative recovery of the infant with congenital diaphragmatic hernia (CDH). The treatment is difficult but consists of oxygenation, ventilation, vasodilators and perhaps fentanyl. There was a recent report where a group of infants with CDH, which required correction shortly after birth, were treated with postoperative "general anesthesia" (1).

The pulmonary system undergoes a transition from a fluid-filled alveolus to an air-filled alveolus. The ease with which this occurs depends upon the amount of surfactant present, which depends upon the gestational age of the infant. Several major happenings occur within the first few minutes of birth. These include development of a normal tidal volume, as well as the development of a normal functional residual capacity. This takes relatively large negative pressure (up to -50 to -60 mmHg), but it occurs very rapidly. The majority of the change is accomplished within five minutes. Blood gases by about 20 minutes of age are quite close to the values that will persist throughout the first several weeks, i.e., PaO_2 of approximately 60, $PaCO_2$ of 36 and a pH of 7.32-7.34.

The third system to be considered is the renal system (2). The fetal state is characterized by the presence of a low glomerular filtration rate (GFR). This is due to four factors: (1) low systemic arterial pressure, (2) high renal vascular resistance, (3) low permeability of the glomerular capillaries and (4) small size and number of the glomeruli. The first two are affected by transition; the last two, by maturation. The fetus and initially the newborn have a very high renal vascular resistance, which, coupled with a relatively low systemic arterial pressure, leads to a relatively low renal blood flow and GFR. This is quite similar to the situation in the pulmonary vascular bed. However, shortly after birth there is a rapid and progressive drop in renal vascular resistance, as well as an increase in arterial pressure. This results in an increase in renal blood flow and an increase in GFR. These factors enable the kidney to perform its necessary functions which are: (1) physiological regulation of the various fluid volumes of the body compartments, (2) regulation of the electrolyte content of the fluid compartments, and (3) excretion of metabolites. The major changes of transition take place in the first 24 to 96 hours of life.

Maturation of the Renal System. Maturation refers to the growth and development of the infant. The changes occur at a slow steady pace. The completion of glomerulogenesis occurs by 34 weeks of age (body weight = 2 kg). After this, it is just a question of growth and development of the nephron. The immaturity of the kidney is demonstrated by the infant being an obligate loser of sodium. This means that the distal tubule is unable to completely reabsorb the sodium that is presented to it even in the face of a sodium deficit and high levels of aldosterone. The infant at birth is 80% water by weight, and this decreases to the mature value of 65% by 12 months. The major change is the reduction in extracellular fluid from 40% of body weight at birth to 25% at 12 months.

The placenta of the mother determines the initial electrolytes and creatinine of the newborn infant. The infant's values are identical

with the mother's. The creatinine is about .6-.7 mg/dl. By one month
of age the serum creatinine has dropped to 0.25 mg/dl; and by 14 years
of age, it is up to approximately 0.7 mg/dl. The question of how to
evaluate the degree of maturation of the infant's kidney has been a
subject of much discussion. If one uses the amount of renal function
per unit of body water rather than the square meter system, then the
maturation of the kidney is approximately 80% completed by one month of
age. The practical applications of these facts are: (1) all fluids
given to infants must contain sodium, and (2) by one month of age the
infant's renal system is able to tolerate any reasonable degree of
fluid administration.

Maturation of the Respiratory System. The infant is born with a
shopping list of respiratory handicaps. These include increased oxygen
consumption, problems with chest wall mechanics, a slow maturation of
ventilatory muscles, a high minute ventilation to FRC ratio, and a high
closing volume. Table I lists these values in a newborn and in an
adult.

TABLE 1. Normal Respiratory Values for the Newborn Compared with Those
for the Adult.

	Newborn	Adult
Respiratory frequency	30-40	12-16
Tidal volume (V_t) (mL · kg^1)	6-8	7
Dead space (V_d) (mL · kg^1)	2-2.5	2.2
V_d/V_t	0.3	0.3
Vital capacity (mL · kg^1)	35-40	50-60
FRC (mL · kg^1)	27-30	30
Resting alveolar ventilation (mL · kg^1 · min^1)	100-150	60
O_2 consumption (mL/kg/min)	6-8	3

The most important difference between the newborn and the adult is
the fact that the oxygen consumption of the newborn is 2-3 times as
great as that of an adult. The tidal volume is approximately the same,
as is the dead space. This results in a need for a higher respiratory
frequency. The FRC is approximately the same, but the resting alveolar
ventilation is much higher so that the ratio of minute ventilation to
FRC is approximately 5 to 1, whereas in the adult it is approximately
1.5 to 1. The practical implication is an increase in oxygen
consumption and an FRC that is similar to an adult means that the

infant has a relatively low oxygen reserve within the lungs so that even short periods of apnea or airway obstruction will lead to a rapid utilization of the residual oxygen in the lungs and a rapidly developing hypoxia. The good news about the high ratio is the fact that the infant will be induced more rapidly and will awaken more rapidly. This state is quite similar to that of the pregnant mother. The high closing volume means that, even with normal degrees of ventilation, there will be closing of alveoli resulting in atelectasis, which increases the incidence of hypoxia. The other respiratory handicaps of the infant include a rib cage which has horizontal rather than vertical ribs and ribs that are extremely pliable. Therefore, the chest wall is quite susceptible to retraction with the normal negative intrathoracic pressures that occur with diaphragmatic breathing and especially with any degree of respiratory obstruction or muscle relaxation from anesthetics.

The maturation of muscle fibers of the diaphragm and intercostal muscles are extremely important. Our muscular system is divided into two types of muscles: Type I fibers, classified as slow twitch, high oxidative; and Type II, classified as fast twitch, low oxidative. Type I fibers, which can be thought of as marathon fibers since they are necessary for prolonged muscle activity, are in relatively low number at birth. Type II muscles can be thought of as the sprinting muscles and are susceptible to fatigue. They are unable to sustain the necessary continuous activity that respiratory muscles need for the long term. The diaphragm of the premature contains 10% Type I muscles; the newborn, 25% Type I; and it is not until 8 months of age that the mature figure of 55% of Type I muscles is reached. For intercostal muscles, percentages of Type I muscles are 20% in the premature and 40% in the newborn. In the mature state, the intercostals contain approximately 65% Type I fibers, and this degree of maturation is achieved at approximately two months of age (3).

Maturation of the Cardiovascular System. The cardiovascular system also undergoes maturation over the first year or so of life. In sheep, 30% of cardiac muscle in the fetus is contractile mass, whereas in the adult approximately 60% of the muscle is contractile mass. The newborn and neonatal resting cardiac output is very close to the maximum cardiac output (4). In the mature state cardiac output can

increase by a factor of 3-5. The low comlpiance of the immature heart
means that increases in stroke volume are limited therefore cardiac
output is more rate limited than in the mature heart. The other
important factor is that sympathetic innervation is incompletely
developed. In addition, the baroreceptor reflexes of the newborn have
been shown not to be fully mature (5). The practical implication of
this last factor is a limitation in the ability of the infant to
compensate for hypotension by an increase in heart rate. The other
physiological factor of importance is that the newborn infant is highly
vagotonic. The premature infant with its immature CNS is subject to
episodes of apnea and bradycardia which complicate the perioperative
care of these infants.

Practical Implications of These Basic Changes. Many questions of
technique arise, such as (1) whether or not to intubate, (2) whether or
not to ventilate, (3) the indications for anticholinergics, (4)
techniques of intubation and extubation, (5) the "best" anesthetic
technique, (6) monitoring, (7) postoperative analgesia, and (8) special
problems of premature nursery graduates.

One of the first questions is whether or not the infant should be
intubated. The immaturity of the respiratory muscles and the
respiratory structures, as well as the anatomy of the infant's airway,
have led to the general recommendation that all infants under 6-9
months of age be intubated for surgery, even for relatively short
procedures. It is obvious that with a short procedure, a skillful
surgeon, and a skillful anesthesiologist, intubation may not be
mandatory, but the conservative approach is to intubate all infants
unless there is a good reason not to intubate.

The question of whether or not to ventilate becomes easy to answer
when one considers the immaturity of the respiratory muscles, the
respiratory mechanics, and the effect of anesthetics on the central
nervous system, as well as the neuromuscular system. The small infant
needs a large degree of ventilatory control or assistance, depending
upon the degree of muscle relaxation required and the amount of
anesthetic given. Controlled ventilation reduces abdominal muscle tone
and decreases the need for muscle relaxants. In addition, it rests the
muscles so the infant thereby conserves energy for the recovery from
anesthesia and surgery.

The indications for anticholinergics are two. The infant has a relatively high degree of the parasympathetic nervous system tone leading to bradycardia. Because of this, most clinicians feel that all infants under six months of age should routinely be given an anticholinergic such as atropine. The dose is 0.02 mg/kg. It can be given intravenously or IM. In addition to blocking the bradycardic response of the vagal stimuli, atropine also reduces secretions which facilitates airway management in the small infant. Any degree of bradycardia, arbitrarily defined as a heart rate of under 120 for infants under six months of age, must be considered as hypoxic in origin until proven otherwise. The three causes of bradycardia are: (1) hypoxia, (2) vagal reflex, and (3) anesthetic induced. The treatment is to correct the hypoxia, give atropine and reduce the anesthetic level. Unfortunately, sometimes the MAC for cardiovascular depression is apparently lower than the MAC for central nervous system depression. After decreasing the anesthetic concentration to a level compatible with a reasonable blood pressure, there is a need for paralysis to control muscle activity.

The next question is that of intubation and extubation. The question of awake intubation in infants always arises. It is the policy of this author to do an awake intubation on any infant who is unstable and needs resuscitation and on the infant who has a full stomach. The awake intubation can be facilitated by a combination of topical anesthesia in the hypopharynx, intravenous lidocaine in a dose of 1 mg/kg, and oxygenation during the period of intubation. One of the concerns in awake intubation is the hypertension that sometimes occurs which potentially might cause an intraventricular hemorrhage (IVH) in premature infants or in infants with altered autoregulation of the cerebral blood flow (infants who have been hypoxic). I prefer, except in the circumstances mentioned, to intubate infants after anesthesia is induced. The technique of induction depends upon the choice of the anesthesiologist. If an IV is present, then anesthesia can be induced with pentothal, 3-4 mg/kg. If no IV is present, a nitrous oxide-halothane induction is accomplished. The halothane concentration is slowly increased to 2.5%. The nitrous oxide is turned off as soon as the infant loses his lid reflex. Then after approximately two additional minutes, time enough to refill the reserve volume of the lung with oxygen, the infant is given either 2 mg/kg IV or 4 mg/kg IM of succinylcholine. Other techniques certainly are equally effective but this technique is preferred by this author since the infant is at an extremely light level of anesthesia and this minimizes the chance of anesthetic overdose, as well as insuring adequate ventilation with oxygen before intubation. The question of extubation is easier to answer. The infant's temperature should be at least 35°C, muscle relaxants should be reversed and the infant should be awake, particularly if under six months of age. The reason is that the infant under six months of age has a propensity to develop laryngospasm with the slightest stimulation. The more awake the infant, the less chance for the development of laryngospasm. Extra time may be required to extubate the infant in the operating room at the end of surgery. If the infant does not tolerate the tube but is not awake enough to be extubated, then lidocaine, 1 mg/kg, is given IV. This often leads to tolerance of the endotracheal tube. The dose can be repeated once in five minutes. If the infant is still not ready to be extubated, he can be taken to the recovery room intubated. The infant should be transported to the recovery room with a supply of oxygen and PEEP and, after an appropriate period of observation, extubated there by the ansthesiologist.

The question of which technique is best has never really been answered. The usual answer is the technique with which the anesthetist is most comfortable. Unfortunately, that technique may not be best for the patient. I think we need to keep in mind the various goals that we have for the patient. These include not only the surgical conditions for the surgeon but also the state of the infant at the end of surgery. The infant needs a smooth transition to the awake state. The awake state is characterized by a return of the protective reflexes of the airway, ventilation and circulation. All techniques have advantages and disadvantages. The major advantage of volatile agents is that a high FIO_2 can be given, and if additional relaxation is needed, muscle relaxants in small doses can be added. The muscle relaxants are much easier to reverse in this situation. The disadvantage is that the infant may still have some degree of depression at the end of surgery and this may delay extubation. However, with experience this can be minimized. The other advantages of volatile agents are that they can be relatively quickly removed and require no reversal. Nitrous oxide-relaxant techniques may not fully anesthetize the infant, leading to varying degrees of hypertension which may have adverse effects on the cerebral circulation. The muscle relaxant should be chosen according to the condition of the infant and the BP.

Pancuronium is the choice for unstable infants with a low BP; atracurium is the choice if the infant is stable. I reduce the use of narcotics under six months of age unless the infant is going to be on a ventilator postoperatively or under extremely close observation. An example of this situation is that of closure of a PDA in a premature infant, where 20-50 µg/kg of fentanyl are used and the infant returns intubated to the newborn intensive care unit. If it is anticipated that the infant will be extubated at the end of surgery, narcotics are minimized until the postoperative period and then given in small intravenous doses at that time (0.02 mg/kg of morphine). If muscle relaxants are given, then consideration should be given for their reversal. Recent interest in edrophonium (0.7-1.0 mg/kg) would indicate that it has certain advantages in infants and children. One of these is that there is a more rapid reversal, approximately 90% at two minutes. Atropine is the anticholinergic of choice in this situation. It is obvious that the anesthetic technique needs to be tailored to the condition of the infant. Critically ill infants need resuscitation and general supportive care. As they show response to the surgical stimulation and the resuscitation, anesthetics can be added as indicated. This may be ketamine or narcotics if they will be ventilated postoperatively. At any rate, a responding infant does need anesthesia. Infants who are stable can be anesthetized with any system which will allow control of blood pressure and the anesthetized state and a relatively awake patient at the end of surgery.

One of the questions that arises is, do infants have pain; and if they do, what do we do about it? Infants under six months of age have paradoxical responses to hypoxia, i.e., instead of hyperventilating, they hypoventilate. This condition is magnified by the presence of narcotics. An increasingly popular technique for postoperative analgesia is to use regional block or infiltration. This can be used for hernias, rectal surgery, circumcisions, cleft lip, cleft palate, thoracotomies, etc. The agent used is bupivacaine, 0.5%, with epinephrine, except for circumcisions when the epinephrine is eliminated. The dosage is 3 mg/kg. In older infants and children, a small dose of IV morphine (0.05 mg/kg) will help the infant or child better tolerate the cessation of the effect of the bupivacaine.

Infants have special problems. The premature nursery graduate has the potential to have a large group of problems. Many of these infants have been intubated and ventilated and are candidates for residual lung disease. Infants with residual lung disease have a decreased compliance and increased airway resistance and therefore need to be intubated and ventilated during surgery. They need careful postoperative observation and probably are not candidates for outpatient surgery. Infants who have had bronchopulmonary dysplasia have a seven-times increased incidence of sudden infant death syndrome. Infants who have a history of apnea and bradycardia who have surgery below 50-55 weeks conceptual age have a tendency to develop apnea following surgery (6,7,8,9). They also need to be carefully monitored in a hospital situation. One of the other special problems that is receiving renewed interest is that of the retinopathy of prematurity. In premature infants who have a birth weight under 1200 gms, there is a 50% incidence of the development of retinopathy of prematurity. Fortunately, only approximately 5% of these patients will develop any degree of permanent scarring (retrolental fibroplasia-RLF). A recent editorial in Anesthesiology strongly suggests that there is no increase in the incidence of the retinopathy of prematurity with anesthesia and surgery (10).

Summary

It is evident that the infant undergoing birth and the early phases of growth and development has enormous changes in every major system of the body that require understanding and a close appreciation of the changes. At the same time, the administration of an anesthetic requires close scrutiny of the response of the patient to the anesthetic. This requires precision in the monitoring of these infants so that the appropriate doses and techniques can be accomplished in a safe manner. We need to conduct an anesthetic which provides the surgeon with ideal operating conditions and which results in an infant in the best possible state in the postoperative period (11).

REFERENCES

1. Vacanti, J.P., Crone, R.K., Murphy, J.D., et al. J Pediatr Surg
    19:642, 1984.
2. Berry, F.A. In: Pediatric Anesthesia (Vol 1) (Ed. G.A. Gregory),
    Churchill Livingstone, New York, 1983, p. 63.
3. Keens, T.G., Bryan, A.C., Levison, H., et al. J Appl Physiol
    44:909, 1978.
4. Wear, R., Robinson, S., Gregory, G.A. Anesthesiology 56:188,
    1981.
5. Friedman, W.F., George, B.L. J Pediatr 106:697, 1985.
6. Steward, D.J. Anesthesiology 56:304, 1982.
7. Gregory, G.A., Steward, D.J. Anesthesiology 59:495, 1983.
8. Liu, L.M.P., Cote, C.J., Goudsouzian, N.G., et al. Anesthesiology
    59:506, 1983.
9. Kurth, C.D., Spitzer, A.R., Broennle, A.M., et al. Anesthesiology
    63:A475, 1985.
10. Flynn JT: Anesthesiology 60:397-399, 1984.
11. Berry, F.A. In: Anesthetic Management of Difficult and Routine
    Pediatric Patients. (Ed. F.A. Berry), Churchill Livingstone, New
    York, 1986, p. 57.

THE CARDIOVASCULAR EFFECTS OF ANESTHETICS IN THE YOUNG

GEORGE A. GREGORY, M.D.

Anesthesia affects the cardiovascular system of young humans and animals differently than it does that of adults. If we are to provide appropriate anesthetic care for these patients, these differences must be understood.

The first difference is anatomic. The ventricular walls of both heart ventricles are of approximately the same thickness at birth. Over the next 1 to 2 weeks, the left ventricular wall thickness increases and the right ventricular wall thins. Neonatal myocardial cells contain fewer contractile elements and more ground substance than those of older patients. This makes the ventricles stiffer (less compliant). During the first few months of extrauterine life, these cells become adult like.

Cardiac output is relatively greater in neonate and infants than in adults. It averages 300 ml/kg in the neonate and 70 ml/kg in adults. This increase is used primarily for growth and development and to maintain body temperature. Until recently, it was thought that neonates primarily increased their cardiac output above normal by increasing their heart rate. However, recent data show that they can also increase their myocardial contractility.

Neonates and infants develop pulmonary edema more easily than adults because the neonate's cardiovascular system operates closer to its maximum level than that of adults. Therefore, neonates have less reserve than adults. Hypoxia, acidosis, excess fluids, and some drugs more easily tip them into cardiac failure.

The peripheral circulation of neonates also responds differently from that of adults. It is less responsive to drugs than the peripheral circulation of adults. For instance, the femoral vessels of neonatal pigs constrict about 40% less with epinephrine than those of adults. Furthermore, neonates and some infants require 5 to 10 times as much dopamine or dobutamine than adults to achieve the same effects (normal blood pressure, normal peripheral perfusion, and increased urine output). If the dose of vasoactive drug you are giving is not effective, cautiously increase the dose of the drug and see if a higher dose produces the effects you want.

Anesthetics are more depressive in neonatal animals and humans than they are in adults. However, it is difficult to prove that this depression is detrimental. In fact, it may be physiologic. At 1 MAC halothane, the cardiac output of neonatal lambs is 50% below the control value, which matches the 50% decrease in oxygen consumption that occurs with anesthesia. Base deficit does not increase. Thus, the decrease in cardiac output is probably the result of a decrease in oxygen consumption rather than a decrease in myocardial function.

The decrease in cardiac output is primarily caused by a decrease in heart rate, not a decrease in myocardial contractility. There is, however, some decrease in myocardial contractility at 1 MAC halothane; the decrease is less with isoflurane. Decreases in contractility are partly offset by a decrease in peripheral vascular resistance. Isoflurane decreases peripheral vascular resistance more than halothane.

Arterial blood pressure decreases less in neonates than it does in 1 to 6 month old patients, but the decrease is greater in both groups than it is in adults. Despite the decrease in arterial blood pressure, heart rate does not increase. This is consistent with the fact that these anesthetics inhibit the baroreceptor response. In fact, 0.5 MAC halothane obliterates >90% of the baroresponse in neonatal rabbits and about 50% in adults. The same is true of nitrous oxide. Seventy percent nitrous oxide obliterates >90% of the baroresponse of neonates, but only obliterates about 10% of the response in adult rabbits. The problem with obliteration of the baroresponse is failure of the heart rate to increase with hypotension.

Despite the fact that anesthetics obtund the baroresponses, anesthetics have little or no effect on the hypoxic responses of the neonatal cardiovasuclar system. They still redistribute blood away from the skin, gut, muscle, and kidneys to the brain and heart. As a result, cerebral oxygen consumption is unchanged from the nonhypoxic, anesthetized state, nor is myocardial oxygen consumption increased. To compensate for the hypoxia, these two organs increase their blood flow. As in the unanesthetized state, hypoxia does not increase cardiac output in neonatal animals.

THE PHARMACOKINETICS AND PHARMACODYNAMICS OF INTRAVENOUS ANESTHETIC
AGENTS IN THE PEDIATRIC CARDIOVASCULAR PATIENT

William J. Greeley, M.D.

In the 1950's the concept of pharmacokinetics was introduced into
clinical medicine by Dost[1]. Since then a rapidly increasing
understanding of the mechanisms of drug disposition has occurred and has
involved into the recognized discipline of clinical pharmacology.
Coupled with this increased understanding, the introduction of sensitive
assay techniques and computerized data analysis has led to many recent
advances in our rational clinical use of drugs. Our knowledge of intravenous anesthestic agents in general, and their use in children in particular, has benefited from these advances in clinical pharmacology.

The objectives of this manuscript are to review some factors which
are unique to the pediatric cardiovascular patient and influence drug
disposition and effect. Thereafter, the pharmacokinetics and pharmacodynamics of some of the common intravenous anesthetic agents will be
reviewed.

In general, there are factors unique to the children, to congenital
heart disease and to the conditions of cardiovascular surgery e.g. cardiopulmonary bypass (CPB) which alter drug disposition of intravenous
anesthetic agents in the pediatric patient with heart disease. Several
recent reports have documented age-related differences in the pharmacokinetics of opioids, muscle relaxants and the barbiturates in
children of all ages[2-4]. These age-related effects on pharmacokinetic
processes are thought to be due to developmental and maturational
changes in body composition and organ function[5]. For example, the
volume of distribution at steady-state for d-tubocurarine parallels the
decreasing extracellular fluid volume occurring with advancing age, from
birth to adolescence. Another example can be seen in our study of
sufentanil where we observed age-related changes in hepatic clearance in
this drug, presumeably due to organ maturation of the liver[6]. Age-

dependent pharmacodynamic characteristics were also seen in these studies of curare and sufentanil. Seemingly, the largest alterations in pharmacokinetic and pharmacodynamic parameters are seen in the neonatal period where the changes in organ maturation are the greatest.

The specific status of the cardiovascular system in congenital heart disease most likely influences the pharmacokinetics and pharmacodynamics of anesthetic agents, although this concept has never been rigorously investigated. Although speculative, the known pathophysiology of reduced hepatic blood flow in some of the cyanotic and neonatal heart lesions will delay the elimination of drugs, such as the synthetic opioids, which have a high hepatic intrinsic clearance. In our kinetic study of sufentanil in adolescents with heart disease, clearance rates in our patients were slightly greater than those reported for adult surgical patients without heart disease[6]. This finding suggests that the specific pathophysiologic status of our patients, namely the presence of congenital heart disease, was a contributing factor in altering sufentanil drug disposition.

The use of CPB is a third feature which influences drug disposition and effect in children undergoing repair of congenital heart defects. The abnormal conditions of hypothermia, hemodilution and alterations of total systemic blood flow rates directly and indirectly effect the pharmacokinetics and pharmacodynamics of intravenous anesthetic agents. Despite these dramatic physiologic derangements, only a few studies in children have been performed to understand the complexities of drug disposition during and after CPB. Quite obviously, hypothermia reduces metabolic rate which reduces drug metabolism. Hypothermia also decreases cerebral activity altering the pharmacodynamic response of any anesthetic agent. The changes in acid-base balance resulting from hypothermia will alter protein binding of drugs. However, the presence of hemodilution has a far greater consequence with regard to the pharmacokinetics and pharmacodynamics of anesthetic agents. The immediate effect is the dilution of the extracellular fluid space[7]. This dramatically alters body fluid composition, and protein binding. Koren et al, in a study of fentanyl kinetics during CPB in children, observed a steep decrease in plasma concentration (74%) with the initiation of CPB[8]. This decrease was due to both the effects of dilution as well as fentanyl sequestration to the membrane oxygenator. We have observed simi-

lar steep decreases in sufentanil concentrations with CPB[6]. The effects
of CPB upon protein carriers, protein binding, tissue uptake and release
are still poorly understood. In an excellent review article Holley and
Stanski have reviewed these effects in adult patients[9]. Until the
effects of CPB upon pharmacokinetics are better elucidated and until
better methods of quantitating the pharmacodynamic effects of anesthetic agents, drug utilization during and after CPB will remain mysterious
and largely empirical in children.

Until recently, the use of <u>opioids</u> was limited to anesthetic and
analgesic adjuvants before, during and after surgical procedures. Over
the past 15 years it has become evident that these agents could be utilized as primary anesthetic agents[10],[11]. In the past 5 years the
synthetic opioids have been used increasingly in the pediatric population, especially in children with significant myocardial dysfunction.
The pharmacologic properties of fentanyl, and its newer synthetic conge-
ners sufentanil and alfentanil, provide hemodynamic stability, rapid
onset of action, analgesia and loss of consciousness when used in high
doses, all desirable effects for the induction and maintenance of
anesthesia[12]. The earliest dose-response studies of fentanyl, sufentanil and alfentanil in pediatric cardiovascular patients have shown
cardiovascular, respiratory and central nervous system effects similar
to the findings in adult patients[13],[14]. While these studies did not
investigate pharmacokinetic and pharmacodynamic properties of these
drugs limiting any pharmacologic conclusions, the authors did show that
these opioids could be used safely in the pediatric patient and the
resultant effects were similar to adult patients. More rigorous pharmacologic studies have subsequently been performed. Singleton et al, in
a study of normal children first showed age-related changes in hepatic
clearance of fentanyl, namely younger children cleared fentanyl more
rapidly than adult patients[15]. Similar findings have been reported for
meperidine and morphine in children[16],[17]. Collins et all have investigated neonatal kinetics of fentanyl in preterm infants undergoing PDA
ligation[18]. In their study they observed dramatic prolongations of elimination half-life for fentanyl (6-32 hours).

We recently reported the pharmacokinetic and pharmacodynamic properties of sufentanil in pediatric patients undergoing cardiovascular
procedures[6]. In our study we examined the pharmacokinetics of sufen-

tanil after a single bolus administration of 10-15 mcg/kg in neonates (0-1 mo), infants (1 mo-2 yrs), children (2-12 yrs) and adolescents (12-18 yrs). The volume of distribution at steady-state for sufentanil decreased with increasing age. This finding is thought to be due to age-related changes in body composition and supports the hypothesis of age-related changes in pharmacokinetics. The hepatic clearance of sufentanil was greatest in infants and children. The adolescent group had similar clearance rates to adult surgical patients. However, the neonatal group had greatly reduced clearance rates, suggesting reduced hepatic enzyme activity or hepatic blood flow. Furthermore, the variation in the clearance rates between patients was greater in neonates than within the other groups. Because the hepatic maturational process is accelerated, variably induced and unpredictable in the first month of life, this large variation in drug disposition is to be expected. Changing hepatic function effects drug metabolism, making predictable dosing in the neonatal period very difficult. Therefore, the risk of overdosing or underdosing anesthetic agents in this period is increased.

Pharmacodynamic effects of the opioids have been difficult to investigate in the pediatric cardiovascular patient. The problems in studying small infants, the technological and methodological limitations contribute to the difficulty of firmly understanding drug effects when correlated to drug levels during anesthesia. In a limited manner, using hemodynamic responsiveness as a criterion, we observed age-related differences in the pharmacodynamics of sufentanil in that neonates have a decreased sensitivity to its anesthetic effects when compared to older infants, children and adolescents[6].

Many of the inducing agents such as <u>ketamine, thiopental, diazepam</u> and <u>methohexital</u> have been investigated in children in a limited manner, where only a few pharmacokinetic or pharmacodynamic studies are available[4],[19-21]. The little information which is available on these drugs pertains to normal children and not patients with cardiovascular disease. While extrapolation of this data to the cardiovascular patient may apply, evaluation of the effect of cardiovascular disease on pharmacokinetic processes are required. In general, ketamine, thiopental, diazepam and methohexital have all been shown to have increased clearance rates in children. The dose-response and clinical use of these anesthetic agents have been reported. In a study in children with congenital heart disease, intravenous ketamine caused no significant alterations in pulmonary or systemic hemodynamics[22]. The pharmacokinetics and pharmacodynamics of the newer intravenous drugs, etomidate and midazolam are unknown in children. At present there are no studies reporting their clinical use. However, the pharmacologic properties of midazolam, namely its water solubility, rapid onset, maintenance of cardiovascular stability and short duration of action may make it useful as an induction and maintenance anesthetic agent in children with cardiovascular disease[12]. Etomidate also possesses many of these desirable pharmacologic properties[12]. However, the recent reports of inhibition of adrenocortical hormones and increased mortality in adults have impeded its use in children.[12]

The pharmacokinetic and pharmacodynamic properties of the nondepolarizing muscle relaxants and their reversal agents have been extensively investigated in normal children[2,23]. Since neuromuscular transmission is easily measureable, the pharmacodynamic properties of these drugs are especially well investigated. These studies have shown many of the age-related differences in the pharmacologic properties as seen with the opioids. Application of the kinetic data to the pediatric patient with heart disease is reasonable, although the direct effects of renal and hepatic blood flow during bypass should be taken into account on an individual basis.

In conclusion, the pharmacokinetic study of the commonly used intravenous anesthestic agents in children with cardiovascular disease is progressing rapidly. Knowledge regarding the pharmacodynamic effects of these drugs is lagging behind due to difficulty in quantitative determination of clinical drug effects. Future investigations of the quantification of clinical effects to drug levels is necessary. In the end, the clinical usefulness of intravenous agents will be based on controlled clinical trials using pharmacodynamic criteria.

REFERENCES

1. Bartels H: Drug therapy in childhood: what has been done. Pediatr Pharmacol 3:131, 1983.

2. Fisher DM, O'Keefe C, Stanski DR, Cronnelly R, Miller RD, Gregory GA: Pharmacokinetics and pharmacodynamics of d-tubocurarine in infants, children and adults. Anesthesiology 57:203, 1982.

3. Davis PJ, Robinson KA, Stiller RL, Cook Dr: Sufentanil kinetics in infants and children. Anesthesiology 63:A472, 1985.

4. Sorbo S, Hudson RJ, Loomis JC: The pharmacokinetics of thiopental in pediatric surgical patients. Anesthesiology 61:666, 1984.

5. Morselli PL, Franco-Morselli R, Bossi L: Clinical pharmacokinetics in newborns and infants. Age-related differences and therapeutic implications. Clinical Pharmacokinetics 1:2, 1976.

6. Greeley WJ, de Bruijn NP, Davis DP: Pharmacokinetics of sufentanil in the pediatric cardiovascular patient. Anesthesiology (in press), 1986.

7. Breckenridge IM, Digerness SB, Kirklin JW: Validity of concept of increase extracellular fluid after open heart surgery. Surgical Forum 20:169, 1969.

8. Koren G, Crean P, Klein J, Goresley G, Villamater J, MacLeod SM: Sequestration of fentanyl by cardiopulmonary bypass (CPBP). Eur J Clin Pharmacol 27(1):51, 1984.

9. Holley FO, Ponganis KV, Stanski DR: Effect of cardiopulmonary bypass on the pharmacokinetics of drugs. Clinical Pharmacokinetics 7:234, 1982.

10. Lowenstein E, Hallowel P, Levine FH: Cardiovascular response to large doses of intravenous morphine in man. N Eng J Med 281:1389, 1969.

11. Lunn JK, Stanley TH, Eisele J: High-dose fentanyl anesthesia for coronary artery surgery: Plasma fentanyl concentrations and influence of nitrous oxide on cardiovascular responses. Anesth Analg 58:390, 1979.

12. Davis PJ, Cook DR: Clinical pharmacokinetics of newer anesthetic agents. Clinical Pharmacokinetics 11(1):18, 1986.

13. Hickey PR, Hansen DD: Fentanyl-and sufentanil-oxygen-pancuronuim anesthesia for cardiac surgery in infants. Anesth Analg 63:117, 1984.

14. Moore, RA, Yang SS, McNicholas KW, Gallagher JD, Clark DL: Hemodynamic and anesthetic effects of sufentanil as the sole anesthetic for pediatric cardiovascular surgery. Anesthesiology

62:725, 1985.

15. Singleton MA, Rosen JI, Fisher DM: Pharmacokinetics of fentanyl in infants and children. Anesthesiology 61:A440, 1984.

16. Vanderberghe H, MacLeod S, Chuiyanja H, Endinyi L, Soldin S: Pharmacokinetics of intravenous morphine in balanced anesthesia: studies in children. Drug Metab Rev 14(5):887, 1983.

17. Morselli PL, Rovei N: Placental transfer of pethidine and nor-pethidine and their pharmacokinetics in the newborn. Eur J Clin Pharm 1:25, 1980.

18. Collins C, Koren G, Crean P, Klein J, Roy WL, MacLeod SM: Fentanyl pharmacokinetics and hemodynamic effects in preterm infants during ligation of patent ductus arteriosis. Anesth Analg 64(11):1078, 1985.

19. Rodnay PA, Hollinger I, Santi A, Nagoshima H: Ketamine for pediatric cardiac anesthesia. Anaesthetist 25(6):259, 1976.

20. Rane A, Wilson JT: Clinical pharmacokinetics in infants and children. Clin Pharmacokinetics 1(1):2, 1976.

21. Quaynor H, Corby M, Bjorbman S: Rectal induction of anesthesia in children with methohexatone. Patient acceptability and clinical pharmacokinetics. Br J Anaesth 57(6):573, 1985.

22. Morray JP, Lynn AM, Stamm SJ, Herndon PS, Kawabori I, Stevenson JG: Hemodynamic effects of ketamine in children with congenital heart disease. Anesth Analg 63(10):895, 1984.

23. Fisher DK, Cronnely R, Sharma M, Miller RD: Clinical pharmacology of edrophonium in infants and children. Anesthesiology 61(4):428, 1984.

PERSISTENT PULMONARY HYPERTENSION IN THE NEWBORN: CAUSES AND
THERAPEUTIC HORIZONS

F. A. BERRY

In order to understand the concept of persistent pulmonary
hypertension, it is necessary to review briefly the transition of the
pulmonary and cardiovascular circuit that occurs when the infant passes
from the fetal state to the newborn state.   In utero there is a
relatively high pulmonary vascular resistance and relatively low
systemic vascular resistance.   In addition, the ductus arteriosus and
the foramen ovale are wide-open shunts.   The result is that 90% of the
blood flow that returns from the superior vena cava and is pumped by
the right ventricle and out the pulmonary artery, shunts through the
ductus thereby bypassing the lungs.   About 10 percent of the blood flow
is used for the growth and development of the lung, while 90% is
shunted through the ductus and down the descending aorta.   The alveoli
at this time are fluid-filled and relatively collapsed.   At the time of
birth, with the expansion of the lungs, there is a decrease in
pulmonary vascular resistance and an increase in systemic vascular
resistance.   In addition, the increasing amounts of oxygen cause the
ductus arteriosus to constrict.   The result is an increase in pulmonary
blood flow.   In addition, as the pressure on the left side of the heart
increases compared to the right, there is a functional closing of the
foramen ovale.

There are many neonatal conditions that can jeopardize this fine
balance between pulmonary blood flow, pulmonary artery pressures, and
oxygenation.   The term "persistent pulmonary hypertension" was in the
past called "persistent fetal circulation."   Persistent fetal
circulation is obviously a misnomer since the placenta was eliminated
at birth.   Therefore, it helps to understand the problem better if the
term "persistent pulmonary hypertension" is used.   Persistent pulmonary
hypertension is associated with meconium aspiration, perinatal
asphyxia, the respiratory distress syndrome, and may occur after the

repair of a congenital diaphragmatic hernia. Congenital diaphragmatic
hernia and meconium aspiration mainly will be discussed.

If an infant becomes symptomatic from a diaphragmatic hernia
within the first 12 to 24 hours of life, this usually signals a severe
process. There are three groups of patients with a congenital
diaphragmatic hernia depending upon how early in fetal life the hernia
occurs and how much compression of the lung and pulmonary vascular bed
occurs. If the hernia occurs very early in fetal life and if the
viscera compress the lung at an early stage of development, the result
is a hypoplastic lung and hypoplastic vasculature that will never be
functional. If the diaphragmatic hernia is smaller and the herniation
occurs later, there will be compression of a lung which will have
incomplete vasculature and lung development. In this situation the
pulmonary vascular bed has very reactive vasculature and the infant may
revert to the state of pulmonary hypertension quite easily and with
little provocation. The third group is where the hernia is small and
occurs late so that there is normal development of the lungs and
pulmonary vasculature. Usually infants in all three groups, even
though they are often in a precarious position initially, do well
during the surgical period. However, in the postoperative period, with
apparently little provocation, the infants in the first two groups
develop a severe and aggressive form of persistent pulmonary
hypertension. Vacanti et al studied a group of these infants in the
immediate postoperative period (1,2). They placed pulmonary artery
catheters in these infants after correction of the congenital
diaphragmatic hernia. They identified two groups of infants: one
group called "the responders;" and the other, "the non-responders." If
the pulmonary artery pressure went up and the oxygenation went down,
the infants were given fentanyl and were paralyzed with pancuronium.
If the infants responded to the therapy, they were categorized as
"responders;" if they did not, obviously, as "non-responders." The
non-responders had a 100 percent predicted mortality rate, meaning that
in the past, without ECMO, they all would have expired. The
non-responders were then treated by use of extracorporeal membrane
oxygenation (ECMO) (3). In a small series treated with ECMO, two of six
infants survived in a group where previously none would have survived.

Another group of infants that the anesthesiologist may have contact with are those suffering from meconium aspiration. Meconium aspiration is due to either prelabor hypoxia or intrapartum hypoxia. When intrauterine hypoxia occurs during the last trimester, there is direct hypoxic stimulation of the bowel with meconium passage. This leads to an infant who has meconium staining of the skin and fingernails. In this situation the presence of meconium in the amniotic fluid is a signal that the fetus has undergone some degree of hypoxia in the last trimester. On the other hand, at birth there may be compression of the cord with vagal activation, and this leads to meconium passage. In this case the meconium is of a thicker consistency and may obstruct the airway. Many reports have verified the usefulness of endotracheal suction for any infant who has meconium staining at birth (4,5). This is an attempt to reduce the severity of the pneumonia from the meconium aspiration. Murphy et al reported the fatal outcome in a group of 11 infants with severe pulmonary vascular disease from meconium aspiration (6). They found a marked increase in the amount of smooth muscle in the pulmonary vascular bed. This signified that the hypoxia had been going on for a considerable length of time.

Treatment of persistent pulmonary hypertension has followed several different lines. In addition to the general ventilatory support, early treatment consisted of pulmonary vasodilators. If the infant is suffering from a reactive pulmonary vascular bed, there is a possibility that vasodilators will work. On the other hand, if the infant has severely hypoplastic blood vessels or those which have an enormous increase in the amount of smooth muscle in the blood vessels, the vasodilators will have little if any effect.

Another form of therapy that has been quite popular is the use of hyperventilation to reduce the PCO_2 levels to between 20 and 30 (7). Often the infants required inflating pressures of 40 to 50 cm of water with rates of 100 to 150 breaths per minute. There has been recent controversy about this technique for therapy; the concern has been that this technique will cause barotrauma and increase the incidence of residual lung disease. Therefore, at the other end of the spectrum are those who are only concerned with oxygenating the infant to a PaO_2 of between 50 and 70 while maintaining the $PaCO_2$ at levels up to 60 (8).

In this form of therapy, 5 cm of water positive end expiratory pressure were used. It is evident from the many reports and the different successes with the various regimens that there are several explanations for the different results. One of these is that the patient population may be different. Infants who have been inadequately ventilated and oxygenated may develop varying degrees of persistent pulmonary hypertension which will respond to early, aggressive therapy. Their primary problem is not within their pulmonary vascular bed, but rather with other factors. On the other hand, as seen in the infants with congenital diaphragmatic hernia, there are infants who have an abnormal pulmonary vascular bed with increased amounts of smooth muscle. They need major efforts to allow their pulmonary vascular bed and tissue to restructure so that they may survive. The question is how to determine which group each infant belongs in without doing a lung biopsy. The answers are not simple.

The new horizons for the treatment of pulmonary hypertension are in the use of extracorporeal membrane oxygenation. This is a technique which requires an experienced and talented team, and there is no question that it is quite expensive. The shunt is done through either a veno-veno or a veno-arterial circuit.(9) The infants need to be heparinized, and this may increase the chance of intracranial bleeding. Some infants have been placed on ECMO for as long as 7 or 8 days and have survived without apparent complications. As with all new therapies, ECMO represents the last step, and perhaps some of the complications or bad results that occur from ECMO are the result of a prolonged period of hypoxia before instituting the therapy. On the other hand, too-early use of ECMO might result in using a major invasive technique in infants who would survive with more conservative therapy. The answer to this question lies somewhere in the future.

REFERENCES

1. Vacanti, J.P., Crone R.K., Murphy J.D. J Ped Surgery 19:672, 1984.
2. Crone, R.K., O'Rourke, P.O., Vacanti, J.P., Haugen, T., Shamberger, R. and Reid, L. Anesthesiology 63:A481, 1985.
3. O'Rourke, P.O., Crone, R.K., Vacanti, J.P., McCarthy, P.J., Schena, J.A. and Thompson, J.E. Anesthesiology 63:A482, 1985.
4. Carson, B.S., Losey, R.W., Bowes, W.A., et al. Am J Obstet Gynecol 126:712-715, 1976.
5. Ostheimer, G.W. 36th Annual Refresher Course Lectures and Clinical Update Program. American Society of Anesthesiologists, p 262, 1985.
6. Murphy, J.D., Vawter, G.F. and Reid, L.M. J Pediatrics 104:758-762, 1984.
7. Fox, W.W. and Duara, S. J Pediatrics 103:505-514, 1983.
8. Wung, J.-T., James, L.S., Kitchevsky, E and James E. Pediatrics 76:488-494, 1985.
9. Bartlett, R.H., Roloff, D.W., Cornell, R.G., Andrews, A.F., Dillon, P.W. and Zwischenberger, J.B. Pediatrics 76:479-487, 1985.

EFFECTS OF CARDIOPULMONARY BYPASS ON THE PEDIATRIC PATIENT

WILLIAM J. GREELEY, M.D.

Cardiopulmonary bypass (CPB) is an established procedure for support of the patient during cardiac surgery, where low mortality rates
have demonstrated its safety. Nevertheless, the uncommon postbypass
occurrences of hemorrhage, hemolysis, leukocytosis, pulmonary injury,
thrombocytopenia, transient neurologic deficits and renal insufficiency
are manifestations of functions damage and morbidity. This is especially true in infants and children undergoing repair of congential
heart defects where CPB has been associated with a higher risk for morbidity compared to adult patients[1]. Since definitive repair of congenital heart defects in infancy is becoming more commonplace, an
understanding of the effects of CPB is fundamental to those who anesthetize these patients. And while the quality of surgical repair and the
preoperative status of the patient are the primary determining factors
influencing outcome, the direct and indirect effects of CPB can adversely influence survival.

The objectives of this manuscript will be to focus upon four abnormal conditions occuring during CPB, namely 1) alterations of systemic
blood flow, 2) hypothermia, 3) hemodilution, 4) blood-artifical surface
interaction, and examine the resultant pathophysiologic consequences
which occur in children.

Optimal systemic blood flow rate during CPB in children has never
been subject to rigorous investigation and is still debatable. Broadly
speaking, the determinant of an adequate flow rate is patient survival
without functional damage. In humans on bypass, clinical data and
experience indicate that at normothermia, flows of 2.2-2.5 $l \cdot min^{-1} \cdot m^2$
are adequate[2]. Because of higher metabolic rates in infants and
children, the upper range of these flow rates are arbitrarily recommended. During hypothermic perfusions, acceptable flow rates are lower.
Acidosis with significant lactate production, oliguria and low oxygen

consumption are signs of inadequate perfusion at any temperature.

The immediate consequences of <u>systemic blood flow perfusion</u> with CPB are several. First, blood trauma in the extracorporeal circuit is probably greater when high flows pass through it, which is often the case during the initiation and termination of pediatric CPB. Secondly, long CPB and aortic cross-clamp times have been associated with reduced ventricular ejection fractions, lower glomerular filtration rates and prolongation of mechanical ventilation occurring postoperatively in children[3],[4]. More importantly, there are rare transient and permanent neurologic sequelae after CPB. A few specific studies have examined the immediate neuropsychiatric effects by electroencephalographic methods only and the results are conflicting[5],[6]. Long term postoperative effects on intelligence function have been difficult to study.

In general, because intracardiac repair of congenital defects often involves open communications with the left side of the heart through septal defects and left ventricular outflow reconstruction, there is high risk for introduction of air and particulate emboli with resultant neurologic sequelae. Slogoff et al have shown that adult patients undergoing repair of aortic valve disease with an open left ventricle have a greater incidence of neurologic sequelae than those patients where the left side of the heart was not entered[7]. While never investigated, the same phenomenon is probably true in children with open left ventricles.

Direct evidence for neurological sequelae solely due to CPB is limited and inconclusive in children. Under most circumstances where continuous CPB is used, neurologic and developmental outcome is more closely related to such risk variables as: failure of previous palliative surgery to alleviate hypoxemia, growth failure, congestive heart failure, stroke, CNS infections and psychosocial factors[8]. With adequate temperature-corrected systemic flow rates in children, CPB is a relatively safe procedure. However, the use of total circulatory arrest (TCA) or very low flow states and deep hypothermia to provide organ protection and a relatively bloodless operative field have their own potential for causing end-organ injury of the brain. The circumstantial evidence for TCA-associated neurologic injury has been intensely investigated. Well documented occurrences of seizures, choreoathetosis, coma in the early postoperative period and late occurrences of lowered intellectual and developmental functioning have been substantiated following TCA[9],[10]. Although the data are somewhat conflicting, TCA greater than 60 minutes at 18-20° is not safe[11].

The renal effects of CPB have been firmly documented in children. Several groups have reported no significant differences in preoperative and postoperative measures of renal function[12],[13]. Baxter et al have reported a 4% incidence of acute renal failure occurring after open heart surgery with a 25% mortality rate[14]. The primary cause of renal failure in their study was low cardiac output after the repair. Significant renal insufficiency has been observed after deep hypothermia and TCA unrelated to low cardiac output[15]. The cause of this damaging effect of CPB is unknown. Recent studies by our group have shown that atrial natriuretic peptide (ANP), a potent mediator of blood pressure control and renal natriuresis secreted by the right atrium, is dramatically altered by the alterations of blood flow patterns and atrial pressures during and after CPB[16]. Although our results are preliminary, we believe that ANP may exert a protective effect on renal blood flow and glomerular filtration during the physiologic stress of CPB.

Other consequences of the alterations of systemic blood flow during CPB further suggest a nonphysiologic situation. As in the adult patient, epinephrine and norepinephrine are released by the pediatric patient in response to the stress of CPB[17]. Marked hyperglycemia has also been documented in children during CPB, unrelated to TCA, age or type of congenital heart defect[18]. Additionally, elevated enzyme activities e.g. CPK-mb,LDH,SGOT,SGPT,Asp AT, have been detected after bypass surgery in children[19]. While ventriculotomy, hyperkalemia, hyperglycemia are known to produce these changes, these studies would indicate that cell membrane disruption due to CPB directly caused the leakage of these intracellular enzymes into the circulation. The potential deleterious effect of these metabolic perturbations on the patient, such as the effect of hyperglycemia on the brain during CPB or the effects of increased catecholamines on the myocardium, remain to be investigated in the children. Furthermore, the potential protective effect of various anesthetic agents on these pathophysiologic processes is unknown.

It is assumed that the use of hypothermia reduces metabolic activity in order to maintain cell function during reduced flow states without producing damage. There is little doubt that hypothermia is the single most important external variable to be controlled during CPB, providing for low flow states, TCA and myocardial protection. Although only suggestive and poorly documented, ischemic injury to the myocardium, even in children, can be produced during the critical periods of cooling and rewarming where care is not provided in securing adequate perfusion to the myocardium. The frequent occurrences of early post-CPB arrythmias and late postoperative low cardiac output syndromes have been documented by our group and others as manifestations of poor execution of the cooling and rewarming phases[20].

Another external variable controlled during CPB which effects the pediatric patient is <u>hemodilution</u>. This requirement is necessary in order to lower viscosity during hypothermia, lower shear rates and permit optimal perfusion of the microcirculation. This is especially true in pediatric patients where deep hypothermia is frequently used and where polycythemia is present as a compensatory mechanism for cyanotic heart defects. The immediate effect of hemodilution can be viewed by examining the dilutional effect of the priming volume of the CPB circuit upon the extracellular fluid space (ECF). In adults, a routine pump priming volume of 2200 ml. will acutely dilute the ECF of a 70 kg (13.5 L.) man by 16%. In a neonate weighing 3.5 kg., a pump prime of 950 ml. will acutely dilute the ECF (1.4 L.) by 68%. This dilutional effect will dramatically alter body composition, oncotic pressure homeostasis, and drug disposition in young patients. In adult patients, the ECF is increased after CPB[21]. The magnitude of this increase is related to the duration of CPB and the degree of hemodilution. Accordingly, this effect in children should be very significant although it has never been subject to investigation. Vincent et al have shown that extravascular lung water in infants after cardiac surgery is increased in those children with preoperative evidence of significant left-to-right shunting and not to be correlated with the duration of CPB[22]. The effect of hemodilution on drug metabolism is also significant in the pediatric patient. In a study of fentanyl pharmacokinetics in adult surgical patients, CPB caused a decrement in plasma concentrations of 53% with the onset of bypass and a two-fold prolongation of elimination half-life[23]. In a similar study of fentanyl in children, Koren et al observed a greater decrease in plasma concentration (74%), much greater than would be expected from hemodilution alone[24]. Since the decrease in albumen concentration was identical to the dilutional effect anticipated with CPB, they speculated that it was unlikely that there was any change in the free fentanyl concentration from the prebypass period. Further studies showed that the site of fentanyl sequestration was the membrane oxygenator. Our group, when examining the pharmacokinetics of sufentanil in children, have observed a similar decrease in plasma concentrations (61%) with the onset of bypass and have observed a prolongation of the elimination half-life due to CPB[25]. Further investigation of the complex effects of CPB upon drug disposition is needed in children in order to understand the pharmacokinetic alterations, and more importantly, the pharmacodynamic effects on the pediatric patient.

The final abnormal condition of CPB which produces damaging effects is the <u>interaction of the formed blood elements with the</u> <u>artificial</u> <u>surfaces</u> of the extracorporeal circuit. Hemorrhage, thrombocytopenia, transcapillary plasma loss, leukocytosis, fever, and increased susceptibility to infection are manifestations of the damaging effects which occur in children. Kirklin et al have shown that the highest complement degradation products, an indices of the inflammatory response of CPB, occurs in the youngest patients[1]. He has proposed that the nonphysiologic effects on blood during CPB i.e. exposure to nonendothelial surfaces, sheer stresses, and the formation of platelet aggregates account for the damaging effects of CPB and therefore, place infants younger than 4 years of age at the highest risk for morbidity. Our study of the effects of CPB upon prostaglandin metabolism in children would support this hypothesis[26]. We observed that the systemic release of thromboxane, a potent vasoconstrictor and platelet aggregant, was greatest in the youngest patients. When compared to adult patients, the release of thromboxane during CPB occurred much earlier, rose higher and was more sustained in children, suggesting greater platelet activation and reactivity. Other evidence for the alteration of formed blood elements by CPB have been examined by Wyss et al in their study of the hemostatic status of children after CPB[27]. They observed decreases in factor V, VII-X, plasminogen and platelets, and increases in fibrin split products and fibrinogen. They found no correlation with these abnormalities and duration of CPB or postoperative bleeding. In our preliminary studies of coagulation status with CPB, our findings and conclusions regarding postoperative bleeding are consistent with Wyss et al; the exception being a correlation of platelet loss with duration of CPB in our study (unpublished data). Investigation of other blood elements in children are lacking, such as the effect of CPB upon leukocytes, oncotic and carrier proteins, the humoral system and fibrinolysis.

In summary then, the unphysiological conditions of CPB such as marked alterations of systemic blood flow, hypothermia, hemodilution, and the nonendothelial surface interaction with formed blood components, exert significant effects on the pediatric patient. In many circumstances, the potential for the greatest damaging effects are in the youngest patients. While preoperative condition of the patient and execution of the surgical correction are important determinants of outcome, the effects of CPB and the attendant complications influence the surgical result. Further investigation of these effects is warranted.

REFERENCES

1. Kirklin JK, Westaby S, Blackstone EH, Kirklind JW, Chenowith DE, Pacifico AD: Complement and the damaging effects of cardiopulmonary bypass. J Thorac Cardiovasc Surg 86:845, 1983
2. Moffitt EA, Kirklind JW, Theye RA: Physiologic studies during whole-body perfusion and tetralogy of Fallot. J Thorac Cardiovasc Surg 44:180, 1962
3. Covitz W, Eubig C, Moore HV, Truman AT, Sellers BV, Shelnutt R, Hadden B: Assessment of cardiac and renal function in children immediately after open heart surgery: The significance of reduced radionuclide ejection fraction (postoperative ejection fraction). Pediatr Cardiol 5:167, 1984
4. Kanter RK, Bove EL, Tobin JR, Zimmerman JJ: Prolonged mechanical ventilation of infants after open heart surgery. Crit Care Med 14:211, 1986
5. Kochen ME, Olszowka JS, Subramanian S: Electroencephalographic and neurologic correlates of deep hypothermia and circulatory arrest in infants. Ann Thorac Surg 23:238, 1977
6. Harden A, Pampiglione G, Waterston DJ: Circulatory arrest during hypothermia in cardiac surgery: An EEG study in children. Br Med J 2:1105, 1966.

7. Slogoff S, Girgis KZ, Keats AS: Etiologic factors in neurop-
    sychiatric complications after cardiopulmonary bypass. Anesth Analg
    61:903, 1982.

8. Dougherty M, Wright FS, Garmezy N, Loewenson RB, Torres F: Later
    competence and adaptation in infants who survive severe heart
    defects. Child Dev 54:1129, 1983

9. Wells FC, Coghill S, Kaplan HL, Lincoln C: Duration of circulatory
    arrest does influence the psychological development of children
    after cardiac operation in early life. J Thorac Cardiovasc Surg
    86(6):823, 1983

10. Settergren G, Ohqvist G, Lundberg S, Henze A, Bjork VD, Persson B:
    Cerebral blood flow and cerebral metabolism in children following
    cardiac surgery with deep hypothermia and circulatory. Clinical
    course and followup of psychomotor development. Scand J Thorac
    Cardiovasc Surg 16(3):209, 1982

11. Wright JS, Hicks RG, Newman DC: Deep thoracic hypothermic arrest:
    Observations on later development in children. J Thorac Cardiovasc
    Surg 77:467, 1979

12. Ellis EN, Brouhard BH, Conti VR: Renal function in children
    undergoing cardiac operations. Ann Thorac Surg 36(2):167, 1983

13. Bourgeois BF, Donath A, Paunier L, Rouge JC: Effects of cardiac
    surgery on renal function in children. J Thorac Cardiovasc Surg
    77(2):283, 1979

14. Baxter P, Rigby ML, Jones OD, Lincoln C, Shinebourne EA: Acute
    renal failure following cardiopulmonary bypass in children: Results
    of treatment. Int J Cardiol 7(3):235, 1985

15. Vengopal P, Olszowka J, Wagner H, Vlad P, Lambert E, Subramanian S:
    Early correction of congenital heart disease with surface-induced
    deep hypothermia and circulatory arrest. J Thorac Cardiovasc Surg
    66:375, 1973

16. Greeley WJ, Xuan T: Release of atrial natriuretic peptide during
    pediatric cardiovascular Surgery. Anesthesiology (In press):1986

17. Isoda N: Studies on plasma catecholamines during cardiopulmonary
    bypass - with special reference to the effects on children and
    adults. Nippon Kyobu Geka Gakkai Vasshi 32(6):920, 1984

18. Benzing G, Francis PD, Kaplan S, Helmsworth JA, Sperling MA:
    Glucose and insulin changes in infants and children undergoing

hypothermic open-heart surgery. Amer J Cardiol 52:133, 1983

19. Adams A, Burns JE: The biochemical consequences of cardiopulmonary bypass surgery in children. Clinica Chimica Acta 93:101, 1979

20. Greeley WJ, Kates RA, Armstrong BE, Grant J: The use of esophageal electrode during pediatric cardiovascular surgery. Anesthesiology 63:A455, 1986

21. Breckenridg IM, Digerness SB, Kirkland JW: Validity of concept of increased extracellular fluid after open heart surgery. Surgical Forum 20:159, 1969

22. Vincent RN, Lang P, Elixson EM, Gamble WJ, Fulton DR, Fellows KE, Norwood WI, Castaneda AR: Measurement of extravascular lung water in infants and children after cardiac surgery. Am J Cardiol 54:161, 1984

23. Bovill JG, Sebel PS: Pharmacokinetics of high-dose fentanyl. A study in patients undergoing cardiac surgery. Br J Anaesth 52:795, 1980

24. Koren G, Crean P, Klein J, Goresky G, Dillamater J, MacLeod SM: Sequestration of fentanyl by the cardiopulmonary bypass (CPBP). Eur J Clin Pharmacol 27:51, 1984

25. Greeley WJ, de Bruijn NP, Davis DP: The pharmacokinetics of sufentanil in peditric cardiovascular patients. Anesthesiology (In press), 1986

26. Greeley WJ, Peterson MB: Metabolism of thromboxane during pediatric cardiovascular surgery. Anesthesiology 63:A94, 1986.

27. Wyss M, Babel JF, Rouge JC, Bouvier CA: Hemostatic changes during open heart surgery with extracoporeal circulation and deep hypothermia in children. Anaesthesist 31(2):82, 1982

POSTOPERATIVE CARE OF PEDIATRIC CARDIAC SURGERY PATIENTS

GEORGE A. GREGORY, M.D.

The postoperative care of pediatric cardiac surgery patients begins preoperatively. The intensivist who will care for the patient should see the patient preoperatively and become familiar with his history and physicial examination if possible, especially if the patient is expected to have serious problems postoperatively. At the same time, the cardiac catheterization data can be examined when available. It is also helpful for the patient to visit the intensive care unit preoperatively so that he/she and his/her parents can become familiar with the ICU and its staff. It helps if the nurse who will care for the patient can show them around the day before surgery.

The transition from the operating room to the ICU must be smooth. Preparation on the part of the nurses and therapists helps make this happen. All monitors should be calibrated and the ventilators preset so that monitoring and mechanical ventilation can begin within a minute or two of the time the patient arrives in the unit. This then allows all involved with the patient to monitor the patient's vital signs continuously while the ICU staff learns what has occurred in the operating room. It is important to know of any problems that occurred during surgery. Periods of ischemia or air emboli may portend a poor outcome for the patient. These events should be known early so that appropriate therapy can be initiated.

Volume Status.
It is often difficult to determine the exact volume status of patients who are still cold (35 - 36 C) when they arrive in the ICU. The estimate by the anesthesiologist and surgeons of the intravascular volume at the conclusion of surgery is very helpful. However, if the patient is cold, his blood volume, which may have been adequate at the end of surgery, will no longer be adequate as he warms. On physical examination, adequacy of blood volume can be evaluated in normothermic patients in several ways. If there is a glove and stocking change in skin temperature at midleg or forearm, the blood volume is reduced about 5%. If the change in temperature occurs at midthigh or arm, the blood volume is roughly 10% less than normal. If the change in temperature occurs at the groin or axilla, the blood volume is reduced 15% or more. Tachycardia may or may not be a helpful sign of intravascular volume depletion. Some infants do not respond to hypovolemia with an increase in heart rate. Others do.

The arterial blood pressure tracing offers a great deal of information besides the systolic, diastolic, and mean arterial blood pressures.

The rate of contraction (the upstroke of the pressure wave) is an index of contractility if no aortic valvular stenosis or aortic stenosis exists. The peak of the pressure wave should be sharp, not excessively rounded. If it is, it suggests the presence of an air bubble in the line or transducer. The dicrotic notch should usually be in the upper third of the down slope of the pressure wave. If it is lower, it suggests that there is run off from a high pressure (aorta) to a low pressure system such as the pulmonary circulation or that there is an A-V malformation. A narrow pulse (small volume under the pressure wave) plus a dicrotic notch that is in the lower third of the down slope of the pressure wave, or absence of the dicrotic notch suggests inadequate intravascular volume. The mean arterial pressure is the most useful pressure, especially when the arterial pressure tracing is damped.

Ventilation.
        Many infants and children who undergo cardiac surgery require mechanical ventilation postoperatively. However, those who undergo simple procedures such as correction of coarctation of the aorta, closure of an atrial septal defect, or a Fontan procedure can usually be extubated at the end of surgery. It may be possible to extubate other patients immediately postoperatively depending on their lesion and their level of illness.

        When mechanical ventilation is required, it is usually because the patient has complex heart disease, congestive heart failure, or pulmonary edema. As in any case of mechanical ventilation, the lowest pressures should be used that accomplish the goals of ventilation. Usually, neonates and young children are ventilated with a time-cycled flow-generator because these devices are simple to use and reliable. Older patients are ventilated with volume ventilators. Since it is impossible to set a tidal volume on a mechanical ventilator and expect that it will be faithfully delivered over time, the effects of ventilation should be monitored frequently. Changes in lung compliance and resistance make it impossible to deliver a constant tidal volume. Therefore, one usually adjusts the ventilator so that the chest moves an appropriate amount and then sets a normal respiratory rate for patients of that age. Then a blood gas is obtained in a few minutes and the ventilator settings changed as needed. Maintenance of PEEP is an important part of postoperative ventilation in most patients who have undergone intracardiac surgery or who have pulmonary edema. This is especially true in neonates. Their FRC falls about 40 - 50% from the preoperative value during surgery and usually returns to normal about the third postoperative day. In the intervening period, a PEEP of 3 - 10 cm H_2O will return the FRC towards normal.

        Patients who have pulmonary hypertension postoperatively are often treated with hyperventilation. However, it is often difficult to reduce the $PaCO_2$ to the desired level because the pulmonary blood flow is so reduced. Of necessity, one often ends up ventilating 100 - 200 times per min with normal tidal volumes. Unfortunately, the higher the ventilatory rate, the less efficient the ventilator is in reducing the $PaCO_2$. On occasion one must give tolazoline (Priscoline) to patients to treat pulmonary hypertension. This only works about 50% of the time.

Unfortunately, it also reduces the systemic pressure more than it does the pulmonary artery pressure in most cases. When this occurs, the systemic blood pressure must be raised with a vasopressor, usually dopamine or dobutamine. One is often surprised at the amount of these drugs required to achieve a normal blood pressure in infants and babies. It is common to require 20 - 50 ug/kg/min of either drug or both. Fortunately, these drugs have much less effect on the pulmonary circulation than on the systemic circulation. If hyperventilation reduces the pulmonary artery pressure and improves pulmonary blood flow, it may be necessary to maintain the degree of ventilation and drug infusion for several days before starting to ween them. Most patients can be weened with intermittent mechanical ventilation.

Monitoring.
       Monitoring is an important part of the postoperative care of pediatric patients who undergo cardiac surgery. However, monitoring should not replace the physical examination and common sense. If the values from the monitor do not match ones clinical impressions, then the two should be reconciled. Do not accept the monitor values as being correct. They may be wrong!

       An arterial line is usually used to intermittently monitor blood gases and pH and to continuously monitor the arterial blood pressure. A continuous EKG is often useful because it warns of early hypoxia. If the patient has pulmonary hypertension, it may be useful to insert a pulmonary artery line at surgery. However, insertion of these lines, other than directly into the pulmonary artery, can increase the likelihood of infecting graft sites or suture lines. Usually, one can obtain the same information by determining the size of the liver. This is a very distensible organ. It can change its size markedly in 5 min. When right sided pressures increase, the liver enlarges. When they decrease, the liver size decreases.

       Electrolyte abnormalities are common in postoperative cardiac surgery patients, especially if they are treated with Lasix. Hypokalemia is especially common, as is hypocalcemia. As long as Lasix is being administered, it is probably appropriate to give calcium and potassium intravenously. These values should be monitored daily and more often when necessary.

Miscellaneous.
       Many lawsuits that are brought against ICUs are due to miscommunication between parents and the intensivists. These suits often stem from being told that something will happen and then it does not happen. This sets up an air of mistrust that is hard to break. Make certain that the nurses and therapists are telling the parents the same thing you are. The nurse telling the parents one thing and the physicians telling them something else is a set up for disaster. If the policy of the unit is to allow parents into the unit while their child is there, they must clearly understand under what conditions they will be asked to leave and when they cannot enter the unit. Document what you do and what you say.